Men and "Woman" in New Guinea

CHANDLER & SHARP PUBLICATIONS IN ANTHROPOLOGY AND RELATED FIELDS

General Editors: L. L. Langness and Robert B. Edgerton

MEN AND "WOMAN" IN NEW GUINEA

L. L. Langness

Chandler & Sharp, Publishers, Inc.
Novato, California

The author and publisher are grateful for permission to reprint excerpts from the following sources:

R. M. Berndt *Excess and Restraint*, copyright © 1962 by The University of Chicago Press, all rights reserved; A. Gell *The Metamorphosis of the Cassowaries*, copyright © 1975 by The Athlone Press, all rights reserved; M. Godelier *The Making of Great Men: Male Domination and Power*, copyright © 1986 by Cambridge University Press, all rights reserved; P. Newman and D. Boyd "The Making of Men" (in *Rituals of Manhood: Male Initiation in Papua New Guinea*, G. Herdt ed., copyright © 1982 by University of California Press), copyright © 1982 by P. Newman and D. Boyd, all rights reserved; S. Robbins *Auyana: Those Who Held onto Home*, copyright © 1982 by The University of Washington Press, all rights reserved; M. E. Spiro *Oedipus in the Trobriands*, copyright © 1992 by Transaction Publishers (published previously in 1982 by The University of Chicago Press), all rights reserved; J. van Baal *Dema*, copyright © 1966 by Martinus Nÿhoff (current copyright holder is KITLV Press, Royal Institute of Linguistics and Anthropology, The Netherlands), all rights reserved.

Library of Congress Cataloging-in-Publication Data

Langness, L. L. (Lewis L.), 1929–
Men and "woman" in New Guinea / L. L. Langness.
p. cm. — (Chandler & Sharp publications in anthropology and related fields)
Includes bibliographical references (p.) and index.
ISBN 0-88316-594-5
1. Benabena (Papua New Guinea people)—Rites and ceremonies.
2. Benabena (Papua New Guinea people)—Kinship. 3. Benabena (Papua New Guinea people)—Sexual behavior. 4. Initiation rites—Papua New Guinea. 5. Sex role—Papua New Guinea. 6. Blood—Symbolic aspects—Papua New Guinea. 7. Semen—Folklore. 8. Bone—Folklore. 9. Papua New Guinea—Social life and customs. I. Title. II. Series.
DU740.42.L36 1998
306′.089′9912—dc21 98-36764
CIP

International Standard Book Number: 0-88316-594-5
Library of Congress Catalog Card Number: 98-36764
Printed in the United States of America.

Edited by Jonathan Sharp.
Book design by Page One Graphics/David H. Nishikawa.
Cover design and production by Jackie Gallagher Lange.
Index by John A. Dibs.

For Linda

Contents

Preface

From January 1, 1961 through May 15, 1962 I was engaged in anthropological research among the Bena Bena speaking peoples of the Eastern Highlands of Papua New Guinea. I had at that time a Predoctoral Fellowship from the National Institute of Mental Health. The primary focus of my research was the impact of rapid cultural change on Highlands New Guinea individuals and societies.

As it subsequently turned out I returned again to New Guinea for a further year of work in 1970–71, at which time I had a Fullbright Research Fellowship and supplementary support from the New Guinea Research Unit of the Australian National University. I was still interested in cultural change. At that time the major focus of my work was on an attempt to introduce cattle raising to the Bena Bena. I returned to New Guinea on one last brief trip in 1975. Thus I spent approximately 30 months working with the same small group of Bena Bena. Although my major emphasis was always on change I did make general ethnographic observations at all times and can fairly be said to have done a general if somewhat limited ethnography of Korofeigu, one local group of Bena Bena speakers. Further, as a graduate student at the University of Washington, I had worked for a time as a research assistant for Professor Melford E. Spiro who was, at that time, engaged in research on childrearing and religious beliefs utilizing the Human Relations Area Files. Because of this experience I was particularly sensitive to childrearing practices and made extensive notes on that aspect of New Guinea ethnography.

Although I did work on language acquisition I never attained any degree of fluency and worked almost exclusively with interpreters and Melanesian Pidgin, the lingua franca of Papua New Guinea. In 1961 virtually all of the male villagers of approximately 35 and under could speak at least some pidgin and many of them were extremely fluent. Only a handful of women spoke pidgin, none were particularly fluent. In 1971 only the very oldest of males could not speak pidgin and many more women could converse adequately in it.

In recent years there has been a great deal of research on the New Guinea Highlands. Some of this has been conducted by fieldworkers who have attained a level of excellence considerably above that of their predecessors. A few individuals have spent longer periods of time in the field and in rare cases have attained genuine fluency in the local languages. Much of this recent and more sophisticated work has built on and extended certain themes in the anthropology of Melanesia, in particular those having to do with male initiations, gender identification, and the relations between males and females. However, some of these recent observations and interpretations are so much at variance with my own that in spite of the limitations of my own fieldwork I feel obliged to discuss them. Hence, this book.

Although I draw somewhat upon my own fieldwork, this work is not a book about the Bena Bena. It is primarily about male initiation rites, gender identity, and beliefs associated with those topics, particularly beliefs about blood, semen, and bone. It also necessarily deals with problems inherent in anthropological fieldwork, theory, and interpretation.

It was not my original intention to write a book about New Guinea in general. I began with the paper, "Oedipus in the

New Guinea Highlands" (chapter three in this book). I argued that the Oedipal triangle was unnecessary to explain male initiations in the Bena Bena. As it turned out this was rather like farting in church. Everyone seemed to politely ignore it. Then, not being satisfied with saying what did not have to do with initiations, I thought I should try to write something more positive. I meant to write simply about what used to be called the Eastern Highlands of Papua New Guinea (see Hays, 1993 for a review of definitions). I wrote the brief overview of the Bena Bena as an example of an Eastern Highlands group. As I began to revise the materials on the Oedipus paper I soon found myself wanting to write about the Highlands more generally. Then, as I began dealing with specific topics such as blood, semen, and bone, I was led even farther afield into the broader literature on the Island of New Guinea. It seemed to me that certain beliefs, especially those dealing with fertility, blood, bone, and semen, were much more common and widespread throughout New Guinea than I would have thought possible. As scholars of New Guinea have for years tended to emphasize the incredible variation on that island I was surprised by the seeming ubiquity of certain very basic themes. Finally, and without intention, I was led to Weston La Barre's speculative work, *Muelos* (1984), which, dealing as it does with semen and bone, seemed uncannily relevant to what I was finding. I am sorry to say that this evolution of interest did not lead to as complete a coverage of New Guinea in general as either I wished or is doubtless needed. Frankly, I became overwhelmed by the amount of time and effort one would have to expend to adequately deal with these topics, certainly far more than I was or am able to provide. Thus the book and the argument are incomplete. I apologize for that.

I wish to examine and question a number of very basic interpretations which have been put forth and are apparently widely shared by anthropologists working in New Guinea. These have to do primarily with male initiation rites and gender identification, and the use of psychoanalytic concepts to explain these phenomena. But also involved are questions having to do with related topics such as sexuality, menstruation, bloodletting, and secrecy. Still other related questions are suggested by reviewing and examining New Guineans' beliefs about semen and bone.

There is no denying that much variation existed and exists in these cultures. Some are or were more warlike than others, some were cannibals and some were not, homosexuality was institutionalized in some areas and absent in others, some depend heavily upon sweet potatoes for subsistence whereas the staple for others is sago or yams, most are patrilineal but a few are matrilineal, some are oceangoing and others have never seen the ocean, some engage in large-scale exchanges of valuables and some do not. It is clear that different areas evolved in different ways (Feil 1987). Among other things, I will suggest that in spite of this incredible variation there are certain fundamental beliefs that appear to be shared by virtually all New Guinea peoples.

There are many basic questions that must be addressed. For example, did different fieldworkers truly see different things or did they see essentially the same things but interpret them in different ways? How much of the purported variations or similarities might be attributed to ethnographers' interpretations themselves? Are the differences in interpretation a result of having conducted fieldwork at different periods of time so that conditions had changed?[1] If there are differences in interpretation are these related to different theoretical predispositions? Are there perhaps sufficient ecological or other differences between groups to explain the differences? Has the gender of fieldworkers unduly influenced their interpretations? What is the real meaning of certain generalizations posed in the English language by some of these fieldworkers?

---

[1] I have no doubt that this is true in some cases, at least up to a point. I cannot help but wonder how much variation might have been found had it been possible for all anthropologists to have worked all over Melanesia at the same moment just prior to pacification anywhere.

These and other questions make up the subject of this book, which, it is hoped, will help to clarify these basic issues and pose further problems for future fieldworkers. As the various topics covered in this book are all far too complicated to be adequately dealt with in a single work I would hope that readers will understand my remarks to be meant primarily as provocative and suggestive rather than definitive. And if my conclusions are wrong I hope future scholars might be helped by this work to put them right.

I would like to thank all the people of Korofeigu with whom I spent many pleasant months. I also thank Robert B. Edgerton, John G. Kennedy, Keith Kernan, Linda Hubbard Langness, Philip Newman, and Jonathan Sharp for suggestions and advice. Ellen Lodge provided a great deal of help in locating and reviewing some of the materials. I offer special thanks to Professor Terence E. Hays, whose astute comments and encouragement was greatly appreciated. I am, however, alone responsible for whatever shortcomings may exist.

To orient any potential reader unfamiliar with New Guinea cultures and to set the stage for what follows I begin with a brief description of the Bena Bena.

One further point must be made. The beliefs and practices described here must be considered as historical rather than contemporary. Most ethnographers working in New Guinea have described the groups they worked with as they presumably were prior to or at the time of pacification. While some of these practices may still occur in remote locations it is surely the case that the vast majority do not. Modern-day New Guineans are pretty much like people everywhere. Those who come from self-proclaimed "civilizations" that have engaged in world wars, mass destruction, atomic warfare, genocide, and other modern horrors should exercise restraint in passing moral judgements on the citizens of Papua New Guinea and their ancestors.

Men and "Woman" in New Guinea

1

The Bena Bena of Korofeigu

In 1961 there were approximately 14,000 people who were said to be Bena Bena speakers and hence were seen as constituting a linguistic group. This group was also considered a census division by the Australian administration. It was not, of course, a group in any meaningful sense, as the various subgroups that made it up felt no loyalty to one another, never acted together as a single entity, and, indeed, were completely autonomous and often at war with one another. The fact is, the term Bena Bena, which was aboriginally the name of only one of these groups, was arbitrarily extended by Europeans to all surrounding others who spoke a mutually intelligible language. It was also the name of the river which flowed through the area and upon whose banks the original group known as Bena Bena was found.

Korofeigu, one of the subgroups that made up the census division, was at one and the same time the name of a place, a people, and what I will here designate as a tribe. As a place it was a piece of territory of approximately ten square miles located at the southernmost end of the Bena Bena Valley close to its junction with the Asaro River and roughly twenty miles by road from the town of Goroka. Korofeigu territory was bounded on the north by the Bena Bena River, on the east by a section of the main Highlands road linking Goroka and Kainantu, to the south and west by a crest of ridge and a tributary of the Dunantina River, respectively. This ten square miles were claimed by approximately 750 persons who resided on and cultivated it. They constituted an autonomous local group, the largest group within which warfare was prohibited, as well as the largest single unit which acted for any purpose and owed no allegiance to any larger body. Prior to European control there were somewhere between twenty to thirty such tribal groups within the Bena Bena census division.

The Korofeigans had their first contact with Europeans in the early 1930's when Michael Leahy, a prospector, and his party passed through the Eastern Highlands and camped near them. Their next encounter some months later was more difficult when six of them were killed in an argument over an axe stolen from Leahy. After this experience they were never again to challenge European might and, indeed, a few months later they traveled to Leahy's camp at Bena Bena and offered him food as a gesture of friendship (Connolly and Anderson 1987:69).[1]

At the time of this contact the Korofeigans were one of the most successful groups in the Bena Bena Valley and had dominated their enemies for some years. The arrival of pax Australiana was not in their best interest and they remained very conservative for a long time relative to other groups in their area. In 1961, when I arrived at Korofeigu, they were still in traditional dress, still inhabited traditional villages (although without the high palisades), still always carried bows and arrows, and still engaged in many of their traditional rites and ceremonies.

As Leahy's interest in the Eastern Highlands soon lagged and he moved farther west, Bena Bena contact with Europe-

[1] For other accounts of first contact between New Guineans and Europeans see Hays (1992) and Schieffelin and Crittenden (1991).

ans developed slowly and was mostly with missionaries, all of whom they pretty much ignored until well into the 1960's. During the years of World War II Australian and American troops were in the Highlands, a few jeep roads were built, and more and more European goods were obtained by the locals. In the period immediately after the war a few European coffee plantations were started which gave the Korofeigans a greater opportunity to become familiar with Europeans, a familiarity which had few positive but many negative effects for them. In 1961 not a single Korofeigan would work for the local plantation owners. Similarly, those few who had previously been recruited to work on the coastal plantations, because of the bad treatment they had experienced there, cautioned their fellow clansmen never to do so. Most of the changes that had been introduced had had undesirable if not disastrous consequences (Langness 1963, 1976, 1981). The history of their contact with Europeans from 1930 until Papua New Guinea's independence in 1975 must be described as mostly unpleasant, racist, and exploitive.

For purposes of warfare, pig exchanges, and male initiations, tribal groups like Korofeigu often, but not always, acted as single units. According to their ideology the Korofeigans were one people and lived together on the same ground "because their ancestors did." There was no belief in a common ancestor, or even a common origin for the tribe as a whole.

Korofeigu, as a tribe, was divided into four exogamous groups which were, according to their expressed ideology, patrilineal descent groups. These groups were also "local" in the sense that the members of each resided together in a common territory in one or more villages. Each of these four groups can be said to have been a corporate entity in that they each had clearly defined land rights within the larger Korofeigu territory. Their members were said to be agnatically related and all were said to be "brothers and sisters." Each of these groups was named and the members of each believed they had a common ancestor although they were not able to trace their precise relationship to him. I designated these groups as clans.

The four Korofeigu clans, from largest to smallest, were Nagamitobo, Nupasafa, Wai'atagusa, and Benimeto. The clan was by far the most significant entity for the Bena Bena. Membership varied in size from few, as in remnant clans, to as many as 350 people. The average size of the four Korofeigu clans, which I believe was fairly representative of all Bena Bena, was 188 persons. Each of them was politically autonomous and acted as one vis-à-vis other clans. Although the tribe, as mentioned above, could and sometimes did function as one for purposes of warfare, initiation, and pig exchanges, even these activities could be more properly interpreted as clan functions.

Clans could be subdivided into smaller units which I termed subclans. These groups were not named, were strictly exogamous, and were said to be patrilineal. Each of the subclans had a common ancestor who was considered to be one of the five brothers who were the sons of the clan founder. These groups did not hold land but they did hold common religious paraphernalia. For certain purposes, primarily marriages and funerals, they could act as a single unit vis-à-vis other like units. Subclans were referred to by using the name of the oldest living male member.

Subclans further subdivided into smaller units which I termed lineages although they were little more than extended families. The members tended to help one another and sometimes built houses and gardens together but cannot be said to have been truly corporate. Members did not necessarily reside together in the same village.

During all of my fieldwork I concentrated primarily on just one of these Korofeigu clans, Nupasafa. At that time there were three separate villages within the clan territory. I resided in the largest of the three, which was called Sapuro. Prior to contact there had been only one large village, built on a ridge top with a high fence made of timber, bamboo, and cane.

The Korofeigans, unlike many of the other Bena Bena tribes, were strictly grassland-dwellers. They had no access to forest lands, did virtually no hunting, and traded with other groups in the "bush" for necessities such as black palm, stone axe heads, wooden dishes and baskets, materials for sorcery, bird of paradise and cassowary plumes, and other things not available to them. They traded primarily pigs and salt of their own manufacture.

The grassland-dwelling tribes were sometimes referred to by others as the *Numuyagabo,* which I believe can be translated as "place of the pig men." Although these groups sometimes referred to themselves in this way, it is by no means clear to me, or apparently to them either, precisely which groups were being collectively referred to by this term. What is clear is that the grasslanders did raise greater numbers of pigs than those dwelling in the bush, a fact which enabled them to obtain what they needed, including wives.

Aside from their grassland habitat and certain minor features of dress there was nothing that distinguished the Bena Bena very much from most other Eastern Highlanders. They were horticulturalists and pig raisers. Sweet potatoes were pretty much the staple although they also raised yams, taro, bananas, edible *pit pit* (a kind of cane), wing beans, and, in 1961, pumpkins, cucumbers, and occasionally other European-introduced vegetables. They had already tried and rejected many such crops, as, for example, Irish potatoes and soy beans. Fish (*tilapia*), too, had been introduced and rejected. Coffee had been introduced as a cash crop and failed and then reintroduced. In 1961 all adult males had at least some, not usually very well cared for, coffee trees.

The only timber available to the Korofeigans came from the relatively fast-growing casuarina trees which they planted in their gardens, carrying the seedlings from the banks of the Bena Bena River where they washed down from the mountains to the north. Split casuarina planks and *pit pit* (a different variety of cane) were used to build houses and garden fences.

Each clan had extensive stands of *pit pit* close to the river bottom and carried it in bundles to the building sites. Men were responsible for building and maintaining houses and garden fences as well as for digging drainage ditches. Women broke the ground with shovels and planted their crops with the aid of digging sticks.

Traditionally, they maintained a fairly rigid separation of the sexes; adult men slept together in men's houses and each wife shared her house with her children and pigs. Menstrual blood was regarded as dangerous and women were secluded in special huts of their own construction during their menses and at childbirth. There were taboos against a woman touching a man's head or hair and parts of his clothing, casting a shadow on him, being in any way above him, walking on certain paths, crossing upriver from men, digging or preparing food during their menses, and so on. Men regarded women, and women tended to regard themselves, as (relatively) weak, more sexual, less intelligent, more inconsistent, dirtier, and in almost every way inferior to men. Bena Bena women I questioned tended to link their acknowledged inferiority (although not very clearly) with the fact that they menstruated and gave birth to children. Even so, as I have mentioned previously:

> . . . these are not absolutely sex-linked characteristics as Western Europeans tend to think of them. Thus, women can be "strong" (this does not mean only physical strength, but may mean many other things—being firm in taking a position, for example, or being influential by speaking her mind, etc.). Women can also be intelligent in the sense that they are said to "understand" things that need to be done, and when, and do them without being asked or told. Or they can be known to be particularlly successful pig-raisers, gardeners, or curers. . . . They can also be "hard," like men, rather than "soft" like women, so as to set out to do something and ruthlessly go ahead without allowing anything to stop them (Langness 1974:192).

In spite of this, men were always entirely in charge of public affairs. If by "politics" is meant the management of public affairs, then men were in absolute control of politics and thus had power in a way that women did not. Male power was validated and maintained primarily through a complex of ceremonies having to do primarily with fertility and involving exchanges of pork with other groups. It was within the context of these rituals that extremely harsh male initiation rites took place. And it was during these times that the sacred flutes, the *nama,* owned by the various subclans and in the exclusive control of men, were played. Women and uninitiated youths were not permitted to see them and were told at times that the sound emanated from a mythical monsterlike bird (the *nama*) that was with the men and at other times that the initiates had died and the flutes were the sound of their voices.

The large pig-exchange festivals known in Korofeigu as the *i'a nama ga* were held when possible every three or four years. They involved giving gifts of pork to other groups that had helped them during warfare, or sometimes in other ways, in the past. Once a decision to hold one of these rituals was made it would be signaled by the sound of the flutes. Men would visit groups to whom they were to give pork and agreements would be reached as to precisely how many pigs would be given, when, and by whom. While these preliminary arrangements were going on people would begin to insure they would have the proper number of pigs of the appropriate size at the appropriate time.[2] This also involved expanding their gardening activities.

Men would begin meeting in secret to prepare their *kafe,* dancing ornaments strapped to the shoulders and made of bamboo, cane, and bark cloth. These large ornaments were then painted in various designs and bird of paradise plumes would be attached to them at various places. The plumes were mounted on springs made of supple cane and the jawbones of pigs so they would move aesthetically while the men danced. Men said the designs came to them in dreams. They

[2] I do not believe that Bena Bena pig festivals were triggered by an excess of pigs as Rappaport reports for the Maring (1968). Indeed, I believe it was quite the contrary. Decisions to hold the ceremonies were made first and the pigs then raised specifically for that purpose.

told the women and children that the paint was the feces of *nama.* These preparations continued over the space of weeks prior to the actual ritual event. At certain stages the flutes would be played, announcing to the world that such and such a group was about to kill pigs and hold the *i'a nama ga.* This was, of course, a matter of considerable group pride as only strong and successful groups were in a position to bring such large ceremonies about.

It was also during this time that major male initiation rites took place. The youths to be initiated were removed from the villages and housed in a special house built for the purpose. Each clan had a special place where the youths were taken from time to time for various parts of the initiation. This was usually a rocky creek or riverbed, well hidden and nearly inaccessible. The boys were roughly awakened before dawn, taken to this place, and made to wait and shiver in the cold until daylight. Whereas previously, when they had had their ears and noses pierced, they were treated relatively gently and even fussed over by their parents, they were now treated very roughly indeed. Their arms were pinioned behind them, their heads roughly jerked back by the hair, and sandpaperlike leaves, rolled pencil thin, were thrust in and out of their nostrils until the blood flowed freely. At another point in the initiation they had a miniature stone-tipped arrow shot repeatedly into the urethra and into their tongues until they bled. They were forced to watch and hold the *kata* (a flexible cane) while the older men swallowed them to induce vomiting. Then the canes were thrust at them and they were told they must learn to do this themselves. This took several weeks of practice during which time their throats were sore and they lived on mashed sweet potatoes, bananas, and water. The adult men who participated in these ceremonies had to refrain from sexual activity during this time. Toward the end of the several-week initiation period the youths were held just outside the house behind the backs of their sponsors. When each boy's turn came he was jerked roughly around and propelled into the house by a shove on the back of the neck. The youths were then told of the male secrets and the flutes and bullroarer were explained to them. All Bena Bena men who discussed this with me agreed that it was exceedingly painful and difficult and they did not regret giving it up.

Most of the initiation activities were conducted in secret. While two men played a pair of flutes, others would hold branches and bundles of grass in front of them so the flutes would not be clearly visible. The flute players followed the initiates so they could not be seen by them. Similarly, when the flute players passed near the villages, women and children were required to cover their eyes or look away.

During the period of seclusion the youths could not eat food prepared by women. Men donated food from their gardens. While a man's flute tune was being played, the donor led the adult males into his garden where they moved in a circle around a banana tree or a sweet-potato mound and then he harvested it for the boys. At one point, women were made to give gifts of food to the *nama.* The flute players would enter the village and go to each woman's house in turn. The women had to stay inside and, without looking out, pass a gift of food out the doorway. A man would precede the flute players, crouching low and holding a sharp bamboo knife. As the woman handed over her gift he would make a cut on her hand and quickly move away. The women were led to believe this was the work of the *nama.* At another point, just before the initiation period was coming to an end, the women, armed with wooden spears, attacked the procession of men as they were returning from the rites. The initiates and their fathers walked inside the group of men so as to be protected by the others. The women attempted to spear their husbands in the leg or thigh. If a woman was successful in this attempt the husband's age mates would shoot her in the thigh with an arrow.

After the initiates had learned to swallow the *kata,* which was believed to be a magical technique to keep them healthy and guard them from the contamination of women, and after they participated in the rites of bloodletting, which were to rid them of contaminating female blood, they were dressed in new clothing and presented to the community as *nehea* (novices). They then had to reside in the men's house and had little to do with women, mostly wandering about practicing cane swallowing, archery, learning the techniques of fighting, clan lore, and other such things.

When the youths were approximately 16 years of age they underwent one further period of seclusion, for about a month, after which they were *yahube* (betrothed warriors). *Yahube* were in strict seclusion for this period of time and could not leave the men's house. They had to abstain from certain foods and prepare for their dramatic "coming out" as warriors. They were given new, adult clothing to distinguish them from *nehea.* Their emergence from seclusion usually coincided with the ceremonial distribution of pork to another group (Langness 1974).

The fathers of *yahube* began the search for brides for them. Usually the father of the eldest member of the age grade was the first to do this. He and his subclan members announced they would look for a bride. They would erect a forked pole in a central place and other clansmen would come and donate to the bride-price. When sufficient amounts of seashells, salt, and pigs were assured (in 1961 money began to be included as part of the bride-price), the bride-price was placed in a net-bag and then carried, suspended from the pole, to villages where there was known to be a marriageable girl. The party would arrive just before daylight, erect the pole in front of the girl's guardian's wife's house, arrange the bride wealth as nicely as possible, and wait for someone to emerge. If the girl's people were totally uninterested in such a marriage they would completely ignore the visitors, who would then shortly pick up the bride-price and leave, often rather angrily. If, on the other hand, there was some interest in arranging a marriage, they would offer fire and sometimes food to the waiting men squatting nearby in the cold morning. It was not unusual for men seeking a bride to have to repeat this performance several times in several villages before being successful.

All of the *yahube* had to have brides before any of them could actually be married and consummate their marriage. If it was a large age-grade and many brides were needed this could occupy two to three years. And, if there was a shortage of brides, the Korofeigans would travel long distances into the bush to find one. Sometimes they found girls who could not speak the Bena Bena language and often were still small. Brides of this type were brought to Korofeigu where they resided with their mothers-in-law until such time as they could be formally wed. As each bride was found her clansmen would decorate her in a new skirt, shell necklaces, and bird of paradise plumes. They hung pieces of pork from her shoulders and waist and, escorted by her brothers and other clanspersons, she would be delivered to the groom's village. There her clan would enter from one end of the village while the groom's clan gathered at the opposite end. In between there was a long path of brightly colored flowers and leaves. The bride's guardian would make a speech emphasizing that they were bringing this bride and they must remain friendly from that point onward. This would be answered by a similar speech from the groom's father or elder brother who would then walk forward on the path, pick the bride up and carry her the length of the path. Helped by her brothers, the bride would present a small gift of pork to all of the women of the groom's clan. Usually her mother would stay with her for a few days to insure that she would settle down and not run away.

The *yahube* were not supposed to see their brides until they were all assembled and were taught to (and did) hide if by accident they saw them coming. Even so, it was a rare bride or groom who had not seen their spouse prior to their final wedding ceremony. When all the brides were assembled a ceremony was held where the brides and grooms (presumably) saw each other for the first time, were given gifts of pork and instructions on marriage, and then became a couple.

The early weeks of marriage were difficult in that the bride and groom were strangers to each other, sexual intercourse was regarded as dangerous, especially by the men, and, of course, the youths were not accustomed to the gardening or housebuilding that they were now expected to do. Eventually they would settle down, the bride would become pregnant, there was a further ceremony for them, and they were subject to a number of food taboos, the most important of which prohibited them from eating food from any place other than their own clan territory.

To be an adult at Korofeigu was to be married and have children. A man, in order to be a man, needed gardens and pigs to fulfill his social obligations and to do this he had to have a wife or wives to help him. Likewise, a woman needed a husband if she was to be a social person with a garden and pigs. A woman might have survived physically without a husband; but it would have been a marginal existence at best, living on handouts from her brothers, having no gardens and pigs of her own, and so on. Furthermore, an unmarried woman was a constant problem in that men would attempt to seduce her, village wives would be jealous, and the situation would soon get out of hand. Aside from a rare severely handicapped individual there was no such thing as an unmarried adult male or female. Although there was little notion of romantic love, husbands and wives often built up strong bonds of affection over time. On the other hand, divorce was frequent and it was a rare middle-aged adult who had not been married more than once.

The Korofeigans, like the Tairora to the east of them, believed that both the sun and the moon were male even though at times it was said the moon was married to the sun. The moon, however, was said to "look at" women and thus somehow to cause menstruation. When a girl experienced her first menses she was secluded in a special room built by dividing the interior of a woman's house. The newly constructed walls were intertwined with bright leaves and flowers. The girl was required to sit on a platform and was not allowed to touch the ground for a period of one month. Women would carry her outside when necessary. Every night she would be visited by clanspersons, sometimes only women but more often than not by both men and women. Several times, in fact, large groups of men and women would congregate near the seclusion house and sing to the girl throughout the night. While she was being secluded clan members made gifts of new skirts, net bags, and other items for her. Her legal guardian was responsible for providing pigs, which were killed, cooked, and given to those who had either sung to the girl, given her presents, or both. Older women, I was told, instructed the girl in how she should act now that she was grown. They instructed her as to how she should act toward men, to be careful with her menstrual fluids, the duties of wives, and so on.

On the day the girl was to "come outside" she was highly decorated. Her face was painted, she was loaned a bird of paradise headdress to wear, given gifts of shells to wear around her neck, and was made to appear as desirable as possible. She was joined most usually by two girls who had already gone through the ceremony. As in a wedding, a long path of flowers and brightly colored leaves was made the length of the village. A platform was constructed at one end where the girls were led to sit with their backs to the onlookers. An elder male lectured the girls on their new responsibilities, told them they should marry quickly, be good wives, and so forth. Each girl held an arrow in one hand and at one point the man cracked one of the knuckles of each girl's hand. This was, I was told, "to make them grow quickly." At the end of the speechmaking the girls were presented with specially cooked pork, and gifts of pork were made to those individuals, both male and female, who had helped in any way. Prior to this, just before the girl actually came out of seclusion, a hole was made in the roof of the house and a sweet potato was lowered through it to the girl, who was required to take a bite of it without using her hands.

While this was an individual rite as opposed to the collective rites for males, there were similarities. In both cases the young people were taught about the dangers of sex, the importance of avoiding adultery, how to deal with the opposite sex, and what they must know to become fully acceptable adults. Also, in both cases the actual rituals were carried out almost exclusively by males.

The Korofeigans did not have particularly strong marriage preferences or avoidances. In 1961 a sample of 60 Nupasafa wives indicated that they came from 24 different tribal groups and 35 different clans. There were no more than five wives from any one tribe except in the case of the other three clans of Korofeigu from which there were 14 wives (six from Nagamitobo, five from Benimeto, and three from Wai'atagusa). Similarly, of 24 Nupa women married out, there were no more than three in any given tribe or clan except for Korofeigu where there were nine (three in each of the other three clans).

The rules for marriage specified only that one could not marry into their own clan or their mother's subclan. In fact, this was made more complicated by the fact that residence itself could prohibit marriage. For example, an adopted child could not marry into the clan, a refugee who indicated he or she was a permanent resident could not, and so on. There was, of course, a notion that when a group gave a bride they should expect one in return but this did not always work out, partly no doubt because of the unpredictable raiding and warfare in which your ally of one year could be your enemy of the next. Similarly, often destined to fail were attempts at infant betrothal in which a man would agree to reserve his infant daughter for marriage to someone. Another complicating factor is that although the Korofeigans were not adverse to buying small girls as brides they were generally unwilling to let their own girls go until they were grown and, in fact, disparaged groups that did so. Indeed, the *yahube* that got a bride of this kind was typically very unhappy and even ashamed.[3] There was clearly a preference for marrying a nubile girl from a nearby clan rather than an undeveloped one from farther away but this was not always possible.

Brides were well treated during the first few weeks of their arrival in their spouse's village. They were expected to do no work "until their new skirt was dirty." On the morning following her arrival as a bride she would receive presents and meet the members of her husband's clan. Her father-in-law and sometimes other relatives gave her piglets to raise for her husband or, sometimes, just for herself. Other people gave her gifts of bean seed, tubes of pig fat, tobacco, knives, and pots. She was also given a new name because the name given her by her own clansmen was taboo to her new husband's clan.

At this time the groom's father asked his clansmen to help prepare a "marriage garden" that would belong to his son and his new wife and would be tended by the latter. These gardens were much larger than average. By the time the garden was fenced, tilled, and planted, virtually everyone in the clan would have helped in some way. When the garden reached fruition, plots were assigned to all who contributed either to the bride-price or the garden. The recipients could dig the mature sweet potatoes once; then the plot was replanted and belonged exclusively to the new young couple. As gardens could be replanted for two to three years, the gift of a marriage garden got the couple off to a good start.

Women settled in marriage involved themselves in the clans of their husbands. They often adopted "brothers" from among his clansmen (but not his subclansmen). The Bena Bena explained this by saying that the women came from faraway places and could not see their own brothers; thus they needed

---

[3] I know of at least one case where the young man was so ashamed he refused his bride and insisted she be sent away.

brothers to support them in case of trouble with their husbands or when they needed other help. Of 65 Korofeigu wives, 39 had such brothers. Of the remaining 26, four were so old it seemed not to matter, four were newly arrived brides, and three cases were unknown. The remaining 15 wives maintained ties with their true brothers, 11 of whom were from Korofeigu itself and the other four from nearby tribes (Langness 1969). These adopted brothers did indeed intervene at times in the domestic concerns, particularly disputes, of their adoptive sisters. Similarly, a man married to a clanswoman of the bride was expected to look after the clan sister as well.

Although my understanding is incomplete, it is clear that the use of kin terms by the Bena Bena was highly flexible and the basic terms could be, and often were, widely extended. *Afo,* for example, the term for father, was extended to father's brothers, all male subclan members of the proper age, to the man who had "marked" a child, and could be but was not always extended to every adult male of the proper age in the clan. Similarly, the man who helped a boy acquire a bride would be called father whether he was related by blood or not. Relative age was a factor so that, for example, a father's brother who was not much older than ego was called *nhogo,* elder brother. Similarly, *tata,* the term for grandparent was also used for grandchildren, and could be used for a father's brother if old enough. And, like other terms, *tata* could be and usually was used for any clansperson if old or young enough. *Ato,* mother, was used for mother, father's brother's wives, father's brother's son's wives if old enough, mother-in-law, and was often used by children for every female in the clan old enough to be mother. There were terms for elder and younger brother but only a single term for sisters. Again, these terms, while consistently used within the subclan, could also be extended to appropriate others in the clan. Both mother's brother's son and mother's sister's son were called by the same term, *nafo.* Their daughters were called *fofo.*

The eldest mother's brother was called *atope,* "male

mother." Interestingly, as in the case of fathers not being allowed to collect bride-price, the *atope* was not allowed to receive any of the goods or food exchanged for his sister's son. When this ceremony, called *yapifana*, was held, usually when a child was about six years of age (and either male or female), the father of the child would ask someone to act as *bahalo*. The *bahalo* could be a younger mother's brother or virtually anyone else, including an actual clansman of the father, if he agreed to act in that role.[4] The *bahalo* was then given gifts of pork, shell, and, in 1961, money. A few days later he reciprocated, giving pork, money, and other gifts to the child and its family. The purpose of *yapifana* was to insure that the child would grow up strong and be healthy. There was a continuing relationship between *bahalo* and the child's parents although it was more formal and most probably not as strong as that between the parents and *atope*. One result of the customs of having someone "mark" female children and adding a *bahalo* was, of course, to extend the network of kin.

Still another sort of tie that cut across subclan and clan lines was a relationship that existed between two people who decided to share a similar name. Thus, for example, a man might take a fancy to another man's child and give it his name. Thereafter they would call each other *apatnigasi*. This relationship could be cross-sexed as well as same-sexed and the two people would have a special relationship that involved mutual gift giving and help. A boy would call his *apatnigasi*'s wife by the same name as her husband did. This term could also be used by the unmarried but nubile girls of a clan for each other.

The Bena Bena extension of kin relationships in this way, along with the various forms of adoption, resulted in a system of relationships that transcended subclan and even clan lines and, in an exceedingly hostile environment, insured that any

---

[4] Mandeville reports a similar situation among the Kamano where, if mother's brother is not available, a local substitute is found (1979:115). I believe this is probably a very common pattern in these small-scale societies with rampant warfare.

given individual would have the kinsmen he or she needed. If, when the time came to have a mother's brother and none was available, one would be picked.[5] When a boy needed a bride but had no father one would emerge. When an aged person needed someone to help but had no surviving children he or she would be taken care of. Although an old person or a child might have been relatively neglected there were no orphans in Korofeigu. Kinship in the Bena Bena was much like that of the Foi and the South Fore (Glasse 1969) in that genealogical closeness was not always the most important element, very often giving way to the actual reciprocity between and among individuals: "For the Foi, one's 'true' brothers, mother's brother, cross-cousins, and so forth are those relatives who are most reliable as bridewealth contributors and sharers, regardless of their true genealogical designation" (J. Weiner 1988:100).

Funerals were often held for elder citizens before they died. This was done to honor someone and also to insure that his or her ghost would not hang around and bother the living. These were highly emotional events and the person being so honored would tremble to the point of sometimes falling to the ground. When a death occurred, mother's brother's sons were entitled to come and demand gifts of pork and other items such as shells. Here, again, the precise individuals involved could not always be predicted from actual genealogies. Funerals lasted as long as seven days during which time people from many other clans visited and were given food and gifts of pork. There could be tense moments if the death had been unexpected as such deaths were always attributed to sorcery and there was much suspicion. Ceremonies were held in which, among other things, a piece of pig fat was rubbed on the feet of everyone in attendance to insure protection from the ghost of the deceased. Some individuals were simply bur-

5 "Mandeville (1979:115) tells of how, among Kamano, a mother's brother was often unavailable to fulfil his 'ritual contributions' to a sister's son and so a local substitute had to be found" (Feil 1987:81).

ied in shallow graves[6] but more important persons, adult males and especially leaders, were exposed on rocky outcroppings until their bones could be retrieved. The widow sometimes carried her deceased husband's skull, and smaller bones were worn or carried by his children. The Bena Bena were known to have been cannibals but apparently did not consume the flesh of their enemies. Not all bodies were consumed but in the case of a highly respected individual, either male or female, the members of one of the subclans would request the body, which they would consume. The bones were preserved, cleaned, and later presented back to the deceased's subclan along with gifts of pork.

This sketch of Bena Bena culture, however brief, should make it clear that they were pretty much like other groups in the Eastern Highlands, groups like the Kamano, Fore, Gururumba, Gimi, Agarabi, Tairora, Usurufa, and Auyana, for example. They had many of the same or similar customs and many of the same beliefs, particularly those relating to initiations and gender differences. The major ceremonies, as is true of most cultures, were at birth, puberty, marriage, parenthood, and death. Bena Bena culture is certainly very similar to, although not identical with, that of their neighbors immediately to the west, the Gahuku-Gama (Read 1965, 1986), with whom some of them intermarried. As Eastern Highlanders the Bena Bena are by no means typical of all New Guineans. Indeed, it is the incredible variation between groups that has long been emphasized. Eastern Highlanders differ markedly from groups in the Western Highlands and even more markedly from lowland and coastal groups. This variation cannot be denied but in some respects it may have been exaggerated. I will suggest that in some very basic beliefs New Guineans everywhere are quite remarkably similar.

---

6 I am reasonably certain that the use of graves was introduced by the Australian administration and was not an aboriginal custom.

2

Violence and Warfare

It must be understood that prior to European contact violence and warfare were endemic throughout most if not all of New Guinea. Indeed, the work of both the first two professional anthropologists to work in the New Guinea Highlands had to be aborted because of this (Hays 1992). As I do not believe it is possible to understand male initiation rites and their attendant beliefs without some understanding of violence and warfare, I have elected to begin with these topics.

Barnes, when comparing New Guinea societies to African ones, observed that, "In New Guinea a greater emphasis appears to be placed on killing for its own sake rather than as a continuation of group policy aimed at material ends" (1962:9). This passage from F. E. Williams might help make the point:

> . . . There was no idea of sporting equality of chance when the Orokaiva was bent on killing. I have already given one or two random instances in which the solitary stranger was put to death as a matter of course. It may be fairly doubted whether a party of primitive Orokaiva meeting a lone stranger would hesitate to kill him any more than they would hesitate to kill a bush-pig. Nor does the warrior think it beneath his dignity to kill a woman. One is surprised at the pride which a man evidently takes in the slaughter of defenceless victims. A certain Pahua of Soroputa . . . accounted for three victims. . . . The first was made on a raid on the Hunjovarehu people. The attackers having sur-

> rounded the village by night rushed it at morning; Pahua found a man sitting down engaged in eating his breakfast, and speared him before he had time to rise. His second victim was one of a fishing party caught at a disadvantage; Pahua speared his man in the side and he fell into the water. His third victim was a woman. Long previously Pahua had lost a brother killed by the Hunjovarehu people and was naturally nursing his revenge. It now happened that a Hunjovarehu woman, sister-in-law to one of Pahua's countrymen, was visiting his village of Soroputa. Pahua was informed that she was asleep in a house, so he stole in, speared the sleeping woman in the breast and struck her on the head with a club. He was not ashamed but proud of this exploit, which satisfied his long-delayed vengeance (1930:161-62).

Virtually everyone, from patrol officers to missionaries to journalists to ethnographers, have emphasized the violence characteristic of New Guineans.[1] This was as true for the Bena Bena as it was for others.[2] The Korofeigans at the time of contact dominated the Bena Bena Valley, having defeated most of their enemies at one time or another. But warfare in the Eastern Highlands of Papua New Guinea did not always result in the permanent displacement of defeated groups as they were sometimes asked to return after having taken refuge elsewhere for a time. It was necessary to maintain ties with at least some other groups, not only for marriage but for trade and assistance as well. Robbins reports, for example, that the

---

1 See, for example, Beaver 1920; Brongersma and Venema 1963; Connolly and Anderson 1987; Dupeyrat 1954; McCarthy 1963; Matthiessen 1962; Meggitt 1977; Miklouho-Maclay 1982; Mytinger 1942; Schieffelin and Crittenden 1991; Simpson 1953, 1954; Sinclair 1966; Willey 1965; Wright 1966.

2 I must admit that I did not perceive the Korofeigans in their everyday lives as being exceptionally violent. There were occasional outbreaks of violence, of course: wife beatings, fights between co-wives, between men of different subclans, even occasional violence between fathers and sons. In rare cases these were serious enough to cause severe damage or death. Large-scale fights between different groups were rare during the periods I lived there. I believe there were two reasons why I did not perceive this as apparently many others did. First, much of the previous violence both in-group and other had been suppressed by the administration and second, I had been raised in a small northwestern mining and logging town in which violence was much more common than in many other communities. It is possible that in at least some cases the reputation for violence might be a result of "culture shock" on the part of middle-class white fieldworkers.

Auyana would not employ ambushes against groups they wished to remain friendly with, preferring instead to engage them only in what he describes as "challenge fighting" (1982:186). Read, writing of the Gahuku-Gama, described the Eastern Highland situation well:

> This pattern of unceasing hostility crisscrossed the valley from end to end, and, not surprisingly, every group had experienced striking vicissitudes in the course of its recent history. . . . Permanent conquest was not the principal end of warfare, so in most cases victors did not take over the lands of a defeated foe; indeed, after some time had elapsed, it was not unusual for them to invite the exiles to return to their homes. But such apparent magnanimity did not betoken a radical change of heart, for even though a period of uneasy peace or an alliance followed the invitation, the two groups were almost certain to resume their hostile relationship in the long run. Enemies seem to have been as necessary as friends for the satisfactions generally sought by the Gahuku. One obtained women from one's friends and also needed them for the prestigious, largely competitive activity of exchanging livestock and valuables. But one required enemies too, for warfare epitomized the highly prized qualities of strength and aggressiveness that brought most renown to groups and individuals alike. It is not fortuitous that the borders of each tribe adjoined those of at least one friend and one traditional enemy (1965:35).

In the case of Korofeigu, their most trusted allies were the nearby Kapakamaligi with whom they never warred. Their most bitter enemies were apparently Forape and Gitenu, both of whom they had repeatedly defeated.

The grassland-dwelling Bena Bena were thus careful in this respect and also maintained permanent trading relationships with groups living in the forest too far away to be considered enemies. They were dependent upon these places for black palm for making bows, sorcery materials, bird of paradise plumes, shell (which was traded in from the coast to the interior of the highlands through a series of networks), pandanus nuts, betel, and at times of drought for sweet potatoes and other food. Trading expeditions were undertaken only sporadically as they were dangerous. It was often necessary to travel through enemy territories and the fear of both attack and sorcery was great whenever one was around strangers. It is clear both from Patrol Reports and personal accounts that the Korofeigans raided extensively, and during my time with them often boasted of how they had repeatedly decimated their enemies. There were many accounts of successful raids, and I know of at least one village that was totally sacked and destroyed with the help of a visiting native policeman and his rifle.

The Kuma, somewhat farther to the west, apparently did not fight over land:

> . . . As there was no land shortage, wars were never fought to annex ground. Nevertheless, groups could be driven away and forced to seek refuge elsewhere. A group that was successful in chasing an enemy out demonstrated its invincibility and the decisiveness of its victory, but the conquerors did not occupy the deserted areas themselves. All groups lay sorcery traps to kill enemies who enter their territory, and a unit running away after a fight left such traps behind. Hostile strangers could not settle when they were endangered by even entering the place. The land of the defeated was further protected by the general belief that spirits of the dead lurking around burial grounds in parish territory are especially inimical to enemy intruders (Reay:1959:53).

It was the belief in sorcery that brought about much of the fighting. According to Reo Fortune, the first anthropologist to write about Highlands New Guinea warfare, among the Kamano, whenever a man died naturally the men of his village held divinatory rituals to determine who the guilty sorcerers were (all deaths of this kind were attributed to sorcery). They then set out to exact revenge:

> . . . they sent out reconnaissance parties with the mission of detecting a payment due at this time from those who desired this natural death to those who had been ready to procure it by evil magic, or soul-stealing, undertaken for a promise to pay; and sometimes the parties out on reconnaissance were successful in detecting such payments. In an instance noted the magicians and their village, having lost one man killed in ambush, were afraid and fled without accepting battle, shouting as they ran that they had indeed performed the magic for which they had been held to account, but that the accounts were square, since the life they had already taken by magic balanced the life lost

> in the ambush. Their imputed clients were of a different clan and village; two of their young men were ambushed and killed instantly, and a third died of his wound; they stood their ground and fought very gallantly in an unequal affair that culminated to their disadvantage (1947:108).

After such an affair had taken place, allies of the villages involved in hostilities began to assemble. The allies of the victors would arrive arrayed in battle-dress of cassowary plumes, shields, bows and arrows, and the like. The allies of the village that had suffered the ambush would arrive smeared with clay which their hosts would then wash off. There would be feasting and then further battles would ensue:

> If the weather was fine and the grass dry, the attack opened with one party firing the grass downwind upon its opponents, following through the smoke and deploying opposite the enemy fire at thirty to fifty yards range. The village huts of both principals were usually reached and burned on the first or second day. . . . The war continued until one party was decisively routed. The victors returned from the pursuit calling the number of their kills and the number of pigs and bags of shell-money secured in plunder. Their women and children received them back with a lyrical song, and soon afterwards men, women, and children of the victors systematically plundered the gardens of their routed and conquered enemies (Fortune 1947:109).

The role of sorcery and witchcraft in New Guinea homicide and warfare cannot be overstated. Van Baal, for example, writing of the Marind-anim culture of what is now south Irian Jaya, says of this: "Every conflict, if serious enough, might lead to sorcery. Sorcery was the ultimate means of revenge. Its disruptive influence on social life is evident; open conflicts may be settled and even when they are not, they are never so dangerous as the insidious threat of sorcery, which is a constant source of suspicion and mistrust. In Marind-anim society suspicions of sorcery are frequent. They arise as soon as somebody falls ill or dies" (1966:679).

Knauft reports for the Gebusi that 86.5 percent of all homicides have to do with sorcery attributions and the "largest single category of homicides is the killing of persons for allegedly practicing sorcery (99/163, or 60.7 percent of the total)" (1985:118). Among the Etoro it is witchcraft which is most often involved in homicides (Kelly 1993).

Sorcery and witchcraft accusations were by no means the only reasons for fighting. Often fights would occur over the theft of women or pigs or other items of wealth. Here is an illustration from the Etoro:

> Taipa stole one of Ailoe's pigs, and Ailoe stole one of Nawa's pigs in retaliation. The individuals who urged recourse to arms at Kaburusato were the injured party Nawa and the *tafadilos* [respected senior men] Mariabu and Ibo. Kaburusato's desire to fight was yodeled to Sarado, and it was arranged by this means of communication that they would meet at a pair of abandoned gardens on opposite sides of a small river that delineated the border between their respective lineage territories. Each side recruited kinsmen from other longhouses so that men from seven different communities took part. The total number of combatants on both sides reportedly numbered seventy to eighty men between the ages of 18 and 60. The prearranged location precluded anything other than a duel between archers, and no clubs or killing sticks were brought to the battlefield. The exchange of arrows largely took place at a range of about 100 feet.
>
> In all, eight wounds were sustained by seven individuals. The injured parties whose pigs were stolen were clearly among the most active participants . . . (Kelly 1993:350).

Not all battles were fought formally as "challenge fighting." Another form of relatively large-scale fighting involved the attacking party sneaking up before daylight into an enemy village, tying shut the door to the men's house, setting it on fire and then shooting the inhabitants as they tried to escape. If this was successful they would then burn the women's houses and subsequently loot whatever they could.[3] Even though having all the men in one house could be dangerous this was still regarded as the best strategy. What Robbins has described for Auyana is virtually identical to what was true for the Bena Bena:

---

[3] H. A. Bernatzik includes a photo of burned out Bena Bena villages in his book, *South Seas* (1935, plate 45), published by Henry Holt.

> First, the men's house was said to be for protection. They agreed that they could be easily surrounded there, and there was also the possibility that the men's house could be burned, trapping them inside. However, in line with their general strategy of warfare, they argued that if they were all together they had a better chance of escaping than if they were isolated from one another. In addition, two strategies were used to minimize the risks. One of these was to build a small house beside the men's house in which a few men would sleep. It was hoped that they might hear any would-be attackers or be able to set up a cross-fire if the men's house were ambushed.[4] The other strategy was to build an escape hatch in the men's house. A section of the wall was built without any posts or frame. Instead, it had only bark covering it and could easily be kicked through if necessary. The escape hatch was designed in such a way that it was impossible to tell from the outside where it was. Enemy attackers, it was hoped, could thus be taken by surprise (1982:188).

Bena Bena informants also claimed that sometimes a secret tunnel was dug from the men's house that could be used for the same purpose. When attacking the palisaded villages men would crawl forward protected by their large wooden shields and attempt to breach or set fire to the high fences. When successful they would storm in killing and burning as they went. Women, children, old people, warriors, everyone was killed. In one account from Korofeigu they boasted "there weren't enough people left to bury the dead so we left them there to stink."

Heider distinguished between what he terms ritual and nonritual phases of war:

> In many ways the ritual phase of war seems more like a medieval tourney (something like the above account from the Etoro) than like what we usually mean by war. Of course, there are sneak raids, and people are killed, but that phase of war is dominated in terms of time and energy investment by the arranged battles fought in elegant attire and the emphasis on supernatural, rather than economic, effects. The nonritual phase of war is just the opposite: short, treacherous, bloody, and with major economic effect.

In 1966 the Dugum Dani were involved in a nonritual war

[4] In Korofeigu these small houses would usually resemble the menstrual huts used by the women.

> episode, which . . . could only be called a massacre. At dawn that day warriors from the northern part of the Gutelu Alliance crept through the ground fog to launch a well-planned attack on the compounds to the south of the Elogeta River. The attack lasted only an hour or so, but nearly 125 men, women, and children were left dead or dying, and dozens of compounds were in flames. Other alliances had been informed of the attack and joined in, not so much to kill and burn as to plunder pigs (1970:118-19).

I have an account of a Bena Bena incident very similar to this in which the motive was clearly economic. Fortunately such large-scale massacres were not as common as small-scale raids where only one or two persons would be victims.

Prisoners were taken only rarely and usually would be either a small child or a woman. In these cases the child would be raised by his captors and the woman would ultimately be married to one of them.[5] As prisoners were so rarely taken, and then only children or women, torture, as such, seems to have been rare.

Still another kind of large-scale battle sometimes took place which involved a much more formal approach to conflict resolution. The enemy lines would face each other on a battlefield, alternately charging and falling back, taunting their opposites and firing volleys of arrows back and forth. The warriors would hide behind their long hardwood shields and/or otherwise dodge the arrows as best they could. Very few deaths resulted from this kind of warring. Salisbury described a form of this very well:

> . . . The only other way in which disputes can be settled is by self-help in the form of a blood feud. Vengeance can be obtained

---

[5] At the time of my first fieldwork there was one woman who had become a wife through capture in this way. The Bena Bena acknowledged that this form of marriage was rare. It was apparently quite rare in Auyana likewise as suggested in this account by Robbins: "One famous warrior shot so many he ran out of arrows. He then unstrung his bow and began spearing women. But he saw one woman he liked, and grabbed her and took her back with him. When I questioned others in Auyana about this, they said that this was never done because the woman probably would not stay and because men were supposed to be thinking of killing during a fight, not grabbing women. They also said that if this man had not been a man with a name and an Auyana 'post,' he could not have done this "(1982:188).

> either by the ambush and murder of a single victim belonging to the offending clan or by a form of ceremonial warfare on cleared battle-grounds. The renowned fighters of each side come to do battle, armed with spears and huge wooden shields, while their clan-mates line up at the ends of the cleared space, their bows and arrows at the ready. The "champions" then "joust" until one is caught off balance by his opponent, and is then at the mercy of the bowmen, who kill him with arrows. It is rare for a war to kill more than one or two men, and after a champion has been killed the defeated clan may flee, leaving its village to be razed by the victors while it seeks protection in temporary exile. Wars are not usually fought for territorial gain, however (1962:26).

In some areas of New Guinea, particularly in the Western Highlands, wars were frequently fought over territory (Meggitt 1977; A. Strathern 1971, 1972). Even so, the basic patterns were similar. Among the Mae Enga, for example:

> Proceedings open with a period of massed chanting, the shouting of insults, and stylized displays of aggression (brandishing of weapons, feints, and the like). Then fight leaders of each side challenge men of comparable reputation from the other to duels. Each pair may begin by firing arrows and then, using shields and spears, fight at close quarters in the middle of the field. These encounters are rarely fatal, partly because the antagonists are evenly matched, partly because they are more concerned to wound than to kill. The duel ends when one man is wounded or weapons have been expended. The champions congratulate each other, embrace, and exchange decorations, which may include plumes, shells and the lethal stone axes that they carry but should not use in such contests; they then rejoin their own forces. . . .
>
> Once the dueling is over, the two lines open fire with their bows, and rapid movement up and down the field ensues as men shoot, dodge, advance, and fall back. Despite this mobility, each side tries to preserve its extended skirmishing line, and each clan group attempts to maintain its position *vis-à-vis* its opponent. The aim of each force is to turn a flank of the other and so expose the crowded enemy to a heavy, death-dealing crossfire . . . (Meggitt 1977:19).

A. Strathern reports that the Melpa distinguished between minor wars and major wars for which there were apparently somewhat different rules:

> In most engagements in minor warfare women would not be

> killed, although they might be abducted or raped by outsiders while their men were fighting. By contrast, in major warfare the aim was to destroy or drive out the enemy; women and children were killed, houses were burnt, pigs were slaughtered, and territory was over-run, at least temporarily. . . . Similarly, in minor warfare the victors would ordinarily allow bodies to be recovered for burial; but major enemies, by contrast, would forestall burial by hacking bodies to pieces, stuffing them with stones and throwing them into a river, or burning them on pyres at the borders of their territory where the clansmen of the dead could see what was happening (1971:67).

Cannibalism was not directly associated with warfare in the Bena Bena, or, as far as I know in most Eastern Highlands groups, and it certainly was not among the Mae Enga, Melpa, and other Western Highlanders. It apparently was found among the people with whom Klaus-Friedrich Koch worked, the Jale. These people distinguished between two types of warfare, *wim* and *soli*. In the latter type was featured anthropophagic revenge (1974:80). The causes of warfare were the same as throughout most of the New Guinea Highlands: "The histories of Jale wars fought over a period of two generations in the Jaxole and Ovaxak Valleys show that among these people the cause of the initial attack is virtually always a bodily injury or the killing of a person in the course of retaliatory actions. Retaliation may follow an offense like adultery and theft or the breach of an obligation such as the failure to provide compensation in pigs under customary law" (1974:76).

Cannibalism in warfare occurred among the Baktaman where it was "an escalation of the war against the enemy, and is done in anger and lust for revenge" (Barth 1975:152). Cannibalism was apparently involved in at least some Eastern Highlands warfare as well: "For instance, any particular case of fighting would almost certainly involve at least two or three, if not more, of the following features: sexual aggression and/or abduction of a woman; destruction of property and/or burning of houses; forcing defeated inhabitants to seek refuge elsewhere; violent behavior toward those who had not escaped; duplicity and theft; and cannibalism" (Berndt

1992:80). Cannibalism associated with fighting was common among societies inhabiting the Great Papuan Plateau (Schieffelin and Crittenden 1991). Bena Bena cannibalism was only incidentally related to war and occurred for reasons completely opposite from the Tanga case. Only the bodies of highly respected people were consumed (to acquire those persons' admired qualities). Thus if a respected leader was killed in battle his corpse might be consumed by his own clansmen. Enemies were not so consumed. The Orokaiva apparently ate the bodies of enemies slain in battle (Williams 1930:171).

When groups were engaged in warfare over time they would sometimes declare a temporary truce in order to escort their women to the gardens. If a war continued for too long a period it threatened the groups with famine and therefore a longer truce would ensue. Even so, during these periods intermittent raiding would continue with small groups of warriors sneaking up to ambush unsuspecting enemies. Women and children as well as men could be killed in this type of raiding, although they were rarely killed during the formal battles, where they could be found on the sidelines.[6] Hallpike says of this for the Tauade: "When a member of one tribe was killed, no attempt was made to retaliate upon the murderer in person, however long a period of time elapsed before vengeance was taken. It was sufficient that any member of the killer's tribe paid with his life, and in some cases the injured tribe was satisfied if their victim came from the general area of the killer's tribe . . ." (1977:198).

In other areas of New Guinea warfare involved headhunting in addition to the more usual motivations. The Marind-anim, for example, undertook periodic headhunting raids in order, they said, to acquire names for children. As in the Highlands survival depended upon successful aggression. Van Baal re-

[6] The best descriptions of Highlands warfare can be found in Koch (1974), Meggitt (1977), and Strathern (1972). Robbins has also given a fairly detailed description, especially with respect to different types of ambush (1982). A rather gruesome picture of a man killed in ambush can be found in Koch (1974:78). For a useful overview of Melanesian warfare see Knauft (1990).

ports: "Success in warfare was a basic condition for survival in this part of New Guinea and the generally prevailing insecurity necessarily led to an over-estimation of the values of prowess and aggressiveness" (1966:756). The Keraki Papuans, too, engaged in headhunting and warfare, as this somewhat sensational account from F. E. Williams attests:

> It is probably true that the Keraki, so often victims of their too-powerful neighbours, frequently held the thin end of the stick; they lost more heads of their own than they captured of the enemy's and felt more often the agony and fear of the victim than the delight of a triumphant victor, dancing homewards with a bloody head under his arm. But there were enough occasions when the Keraki war-party, after due performance of preliminary magic, sallied forth on the raid. There was the gathering of allies; the secret approach through one of those wide barren no-man's-lands which separate Morehead villages; the fireless camp within striking distance of the enemy; the spying about the gardens; and the final swoop at dawn, when the victims sprang up terrified and confused from their sleep to fly into the bush or fall into the hands of the raiders. Then followed the clubbing and beheading, and the raiders returned with all possible speed until, having put a safe distance between themselves and immediate retaliation, they could afford to enjoy their triumph. Nearing home they moved in a solemn dance accompanied by the shell trumpet, the fortunate ones swinging from side to side the heads they had captured. Thus they were welcomed by the women, who held out their fish-nets to catch the spoils of the raid. Then there ensued a period of rejoicing and feasting (though not of cannibalism except for morsels, such as eyeballs or snippets from the cheek); and when the warriors had recovered from this they could resume their ordinary life until they were raided in turn and lost some of their own heads (1936:26).

Headhunting was widespread among the Asmat peoples of what was formerly Netherlands New Guinea (Saulnier 1963).

Warfare was apparently more restricted in some areas than others, as Fortune reported for Arapesh and their neighbors:

> [In] Arapesh warfare . . . the men of different localities were frequently on an explicit offensive and defensive in regard to their exclusive rights in women. . . . Land was little disputed, but, instead, more readily transferable goods. This broad characteristic of Arapesh warfare is not uncommon in the area. Neighbouring tribes of headhunters do not directly dispute the

> exclusive exploitation rights to land which they maintain. Their offensive takes heads, which are also more readily transferable than land. They remain content with their accessions of enemy heads, and, for lack of an expansionist policy, even become disgruntled if neighbouring areas become depopulated of heads. . . . Without hypothesis, it is clear that Arapesh culture did not promote warfare to any vicious extreme. Warfare was made dependent upon women's sexual consent in extramarital liaisons outside locality borders, and it was regarded with considerable distaste. The chances for domestic peace, and for consequent peace abroad, were very high, and compare more than favourably with the chances for peace in other societies (1932:24).

It is difficult to say with certainty just how many deaths resulted from warfare in different areas. Barth says for the Baktaman: "Life before pacification was very profoundly affected by the continual threat and frequent perpetration of violence between people . . . of the 54 deaths that have taken place from infancy until pacification in the sibling groups of the present adult generation, 18 were killed in warfare. This is a reasonable indication that in the pre-contact times, one person in every three died a violent death. Every live man carries the scars and marks of battle, especially from arrow-wounds; every person seems to have experienced pursuit and frantic flight, etc." (1975:145).

Here is one Bena Bena woman's memories of this (Langness fieldnotes):

> When I was little there was a fight and I saw it. Mehenabo, Netasirupa and Fore came before to fight us (Sirupa). Some other places, too, I think, but I don't remember well. My father fought then and he won the fight. Then later they came to fight us. They came and encircled our place and set fire to the houses. The whites were at the Bena then, when they came and burned out houses. A policeboy came with them and stood outside and when the men tried to get out he shot them with cartridges. I think they had given him a pig or something to get him to come and help them. I was like Gibigie (her daughter, about eight). They had just pierced my nose and I was there when they came to burn our houses. They surrounded the men's house and some of the other houses. There was a big circle of men around the house and I crawled out between a man's legs and ran away and hid in the kunai [grass]. It was

> still dark when I crawled through his legs. He didn't see me. I just crawled out through his legs and ran away. If he had seen me he would have killed me. Before my father had fought and beaten these people and then later they came and burned our houses. Before my father had been shot in the hand. I was sleeping in another house. I didn't see my father and I just ran away and hid in a cave. After all the enemies had left I went back. All the houses were burned, all the women's houses and men's houses. Lots of people were burned to death. We got some water and washed them. They died in the fire and we washed them. We took their bodies out of the ashes. Later we buried them. Lots of people were killed. We went to another place where there were lots of trees and we made new houses fast.

Things were not much different for the Maring:

> Not all fights ended in truces, however; it sometimes happened that one side was routed. The victors, in such instances, after killing every man, woman, and child unfortunate enough to be caught, laid waste the territory of the vanquished. After the defeat of the Tsembaga in 1953, the Kundagai tore up the Tsembaga gardens, cut down most of the *pandanus* and *ambiam* (*Gnetum gnemon*) groves, desecrated the *raku*, the burial places where pig sacrifices are made, burned the houses, and killed all the adolescent and adult pigs. Their depredations were directed toward making it as difficult as possible for the Tsembaga to return to their own territory, rather than toward the acquisition of booty. Since the Tsembaga were *cenay yu*, or formal enemies, to them, foodstuffs grown by the Tsembaga were supernaturally proscribed. Their booty was therefore limited to baby pigs, which could be taken home to be raised, and perhaps to wealth objects, such as plumes and shells, which the fleeing Tsembaga had left behind. The slain pigs were not allowed to rot, however. Neutrals, seeing the smoke of the burning Tsembaga houses, immediately came and carried the carcasses back to their own houses for cooking (Rappaport 1968:143).

Gardner and Heider have given us an excellent account of raiding and warfare among the Dugum Dani and have described the difference between the two enterprises in their book, *Gardens of War*. What they say of Dani warriors is perhaps true of many other New Guineans although I believe it greatly oversimplifies reality: "The Dani fight because they want to and because it is necessary. They do not enter into battle in order to put an end to fighting. They do not envisage the end of fighting any more than the end of gardening or of ghosts. Nor do they fight in order to annex land or to dominate people. The Dani are warriors because they have wanted to be since boyhood, not because they are persuaded by political arguments or their own sentimental or patriotic feelings. They are ready to fight whenever their leaders decide to do so" (1968:135).

Whether this statement is absolutely true is open to question but there is no doubt that violence was widespread in New Guinea and can be seen in activities not directly associated with warfare and raiding. Children among the Bena Bena and most other Highland groups are taught to be violent and aggressive. Boys are especially encouraged in this respect. Play is rough and unsupervised, and the weak suffer the strong. There is no "underdog" or sense of "fair play," as Western Europeans conceive of them. Tiny boys are sometimes given sticks and encouraged to attack girls, which they do much to the amusement of adults. The ideal is to be brave and strong enough to have a "name." That is, to become a warrior. When one is small this is often achieved at the expense of animals which are beaten, stoned, kicked, shot at with play arrows, and tormented unmercifully. When in mourning people often cut off the finger joints of small girls and often mutilate themselves in the same way. Initiation rites for both boys and girls can involve exeedingly painful treatments: thrusting sharp leaves up the initiates' noses, bleeding their penes, piercing their septums, and so on.

Violence against wives was and often still is common. For example, although among Kapauku "an ideal husband . . . should not punish his wife physically—a reprimand should be his harshest treatment," nonetheless a man may punish his wife, "even by wounding her or, for a serious offense such as adultery, by killing her . . ."(Pospisil 1958:57). Violence toward wives appears to have been more common among the Maring, but some men were believed to be exceptions (Lowman-Vayda 1968). In the Bena Bena clan I worked in approximately half of the men were known to be wife beaters but the violent punishments for women described by Read (1952, 1955) among the nearby Gahuku-Gama would have been most unusual. The following, from Mendi, I believe would not have happened at all: "This kind of economic pressure obviously leads to a form of blackmail, with the wife threatening to go home unless the husband makes repeated payments to her kin. This is, however, a risky game—a form of 'brinksmanship' which balances the respective political influences of the wife's and the husband's kin groups. If the wife loses, her husband may kill her publicly with a red-hot stone in her vagina; I know of two cases in which this did in fact happen" (Ryan 1969:173).

Some men had reputations for violence that went far beyond the ordinary. Here is a report for the Grand Valley Dani:

> But in the Hisaro clans to the southward there is a kain (war leader) who is said to have taken more than one hundred lives. He is notorious throughout the valley, even among tribes like the Kurelu which have no contact with his own. In the course of an ordinary lifetime of tribal wars and raids it would not be possible to kill one hundred people, but this kain is not an ordinary man. A fanatic warrior in battle, he prowls as well on solitary raids into the countries of his enemies, killing quietly where chance offers. On one occasion he accosted a woman on a lonely path: the woman, assuming the stranger was bent on rape, lay down philosophically to receive him. His spear lay beside them, and, instead of raping her, he drove the spear inside her. Another time he entered the sili at midday, when only old women, infants, and sick people would be about. A sick boy in the pilai invited him to rest himself in the loft above until the men might return; when both had climbed into the darkness, the stranger strangled his young host and took his leave.
>
> Despite the number of enemies to his credit, this man's need to take life is unfamiliar to the Dani and makes even his own people uneasy. The criminality of his acts is recognized: unlike Wereklowe, he is despised as well as feared (Matthieson 1962:103).

The case of Matato of the Tairora is somewhat similar:

> No one doubts that Matato liked to kill, nor that killing was nearly always on his mind. To those who feel they knew Matato, the very question would seem simple. If this was not in fact his nature, therefore, he played his role superlatively for he succeeded in convincing those around him that he killed for pure pleasure, or simply because it was innate in him to do so. Spotting a visitor in the village he would become agitated, demanding to know of a kinsman, 'Who is that? Let me kill him!' A local style of story-telling, to be sure, makes words of a man's supposed thoughts. Word or thought, however, modern informants believe Matato's killer-lust was insatiable and depict his contemporaries as constantly concerned to restrain him (Watson 1971: 235).

The above two cases are perhaps extreme examples of what Read described as "strong" men:

> . . . the stereotype of the "strong" man may be described as a person who is both assertive and aggressive. He is preeminently a warrior, a man who is quick to take offence, to suspect a slight or injury and likely to resort to force. He is a "hard" man, a proud man, an individual who is not likely to defer to others, a person who tends to act precipitately. He expects obedience, is motivated by a desire to dominate and cannot abide opposition. He is an individual who easily feels threatened by the quality of "strength" in others. Such a man may be admired for his abilities. He will "earn a name," even attract adherents; but he is unlikely to achieve generalized authority or lasting influence (1959:433).

Read goes on to argue that to achieve generalized authority and maintain it one must balance the value of "equivalence" with "strength." While this is no doubt correct, the problem in many New Guinea societies was the absence of any mechanism other than violence to assure that leaders will not abuse their power. As Berndt put it: ". . . a really strong man, in spite of what deeds he perpetrated, could get away with almost anything—until another, more powerful, person appeared on the scene" (1992:81).[7]

Leadership is so little developed in some societies that men are believed to be able to speak only for themselves. Burridge writes of the Tangu: "Experience of the administration has

[7] See also Berndt 1962; Brown 1963, 1971.

given Tangu some further understanding of hygiene and cleanliness, and it is accustoming them to that delegation of authority so necessary to being in the greater political community. But in present circumstances Tangu find it difficult to abandon the idea that in practice a man speaks only for himself and perhaps his wife and younger children" (1969:34).

What Lawrence writes of "big men" among the Garia is very similar to many other New Guinea societies: "Yet the authority of these 'big men' is limited. In the first place, it is restricted almost entirely to setting in motion the above routine activities. The leaders direct stages by which gardens are made. They impose food and sex taboos on novices during initiation. They supervise young men in sorcery training. But they are not hereditary or titular office bearers and they are unable to adjudicate or coerce. Although they use their influence in disputes as far as they dare, they cannot give binding decisions or judgments, and their only guarantee of obedience from their followers is the willingness of the latter to co-operate" (1971:80).

Among the Abelam it is entrepreneurship which leads to leadership:

> The big man of the founding clan is also the big man of the hamlet and is sometimes called *kumbu-ndu, kumbu* being the term applied to the tip of a yam or the top of a tree—the growing point. In an earlier article I took over the Araphesh phrase of "trunk-man" for such a person, but entrepreneur is closer to the Abelam concept. He is sometimes spoken of as the "owner" of the house-tamberan and slit-gongs of his hamlet; and when an old house-tamberan is demolished, he has the right to utilize parts of the painted facade as a front wall for his yam storehouse. His authority rests on his status in his own clan, his moral reputation, his age, his achievements, his willingness to accept onerous responsibility, and his proven capacity for leadership. He cannot command force to secure compliance with his orders; but, once he has obtained the support of other elders for a project, he directs and supervises proceedings . . . (Kaberry 1971:52).

Although the qualities for leadership varied somewhat in

New Guinea there are few places where leadership did not have to be acquired in some way rather than being automatically bestowed because of birth or clan or whatever. Most everywhere leaders attained their positions through superior knowledge or wisdom or success in battle or in gardening or all of these. There was always a potential for abuse and rarely were there effective methods other than force for dealing with abuse. It would appear that the New Guinea reputation for violence was in the majority of cases well founded. And there can be little doubt that violence of all kinds was much more commonplace prior to European contact than subsequently. Indeed, Knauft in an interesting review of Melanesian warfare has argued that the level of violence aboriginally and at the time of contact was actually minimized in the literature because of missionary attitudes and the emphasis on functional interpretations by the earliest anthropologists in the area (1990).

As I said at the beginning of this chapter, it would be extremely difficult to make sense of male initiations in New Guinea and many of the beliefs associated with them without some knowledge of the patterns of violence, raiding, and warring that were so ubiquitous.

> For the purpose of understanding the "male fertility complex," the relevant implication of the inseparability of gifts from blows is this: the real masters of social bonding in tribal systems are those in a position to command both. Only the war-makers can agree to the peace. Thus control of exchange has as one of its preconditions the monopolization of violence. At the same time, peace cannot be made with nothing. Thus another precondition for the control of exchange is regular access to and command of desired items. What is finally required in any system of reciprocity are ways to effect the mobilization and coordination of responses. These ways, differently developed in different systems, are themselves instruments of power, perhaps the most crucial, and it is through them that systems of reciprocity become, always to some degree, systems of domination (Whitehead 1986a:279).

Let us now consider the "male fertility complex" and its attendant rites and explanations.

3

Oedipus in Bena Bena?[1]

There have been a variety of attempts to explain male initiation rites, gender conflict, and other related aspects of Melanesian behavior. As Gelber has recently pointed out: "Explanations have been offered in terms of ecological relations, population regulation, economy, social structure, warfare, psychology, and belief systems, and sometimes in combinations of these" (1986:3). Her own explanation for the "antagonism toward women," as well as most of the other explanations she reviews, are flawed by what I take to be at best gross oversimplifications or exaggerations and at worst by claims that are simply false. For example, pigs in the New Guinea Highlands are not produced "entirely by women" (Gelber 1986:21). Older men are not ordinarily in serious competition for women (1986:19) and are, indeed, responsible for seeing to it that younger men get brides. The contribution of men to production is not merely "seasonal" and "limited to clearing the land of large trees, constructing fences, and in some cases raising a few minor crops, usually in tree form, which require little tending" (1986:19–20).

[1] An earlier version of this chapter was published in *Ethos*, Vol. 18, No. 4., pp. 387–406, 1990.

Furthermore, I do not believe that women are "exploited" by males to anywhere near the extent Gelber and others would have us believe.[2] In any case, one of my hopes for this book is that it will help draw attention to these kind of problems. As one of the major types of explanation for male initiation rites and the related antagonism between the sexes is derived from psychoanalytic theory, this is perhaps the best place to begin. In this chapter I will concentrate primarily on questions having to do with mother-son ties, sex and gender, the position of fathers, and the duties of males and females in general.

In the concluding chapter to his stimulating book, *Oedipus in the Trobriands*, when speaking of male initiation rites, particularly in New Guinea, Melford Spiro makes the following statement: "I must hasten to say, however, that an Oedipal interpretation of these rites not only is *not* obvious to other commentators, but has typically been rejected by anthropologists (see Langness 1974) and psychoanalysts (see Lidz and Lidz 1977) alike" (1982:169).

In the 1974 paper referred to I had discussed male initiation rites among the Bena Bena and suggested it was not necessary to posit Oedipal conflict as part of the explanation (1974:210).

Spiro then goes on to discuss the "blatant" Oedipal meanings Gilbert Herdt has unearthed for the Sambia (Herdt 1981),

---

[2] In his fine work on *The Evolution of Highland Papua New Guinea Societies* Feil says: "Aggressive masculinity in the Eastern Highlands, apparently so vulnerable and fragile, is bolstered by an ideology which consistently and uncompromisingly proclaims male ascendancy, and accompanying social practice which isolates, denigrates, and completely subordinates women" (1987:124). And then again, "Men could never be seen to be weak or soft in dealings with women. This strident misogyny, of pathological proportions, is nowhere so manifest in the highlands as here [Gahuku-Gama]. Sexual antagonism is fundamental, inherent, and, like warfare in the eastern highlands, unrestricted. Men do not require specific incidents or reasons to abuse or mistreat women; it is part of the normal course of events; indeed, in ritual and myth, it is portrayed as the essential order of things" (1987:203). I would suggest that this type of behavior is portrayed in myth and ritual far more than it actually appears in the daily lives of Eastern Highlanders. I believe these are exceedingly strong overstatements based upon a history of such claims and exaggerations that appear in the literature on the Eastern Highlands. I hope this will become clearer as we proceed.

citing in some detail the various brutal practices engaged in during Sambia initiations. Michael Allen, in his book on male cults, had previously suggested there might be cases where male initiations were practiced but no Oedipal rivalry was involved (1967:22). Allen suggested that:

> Male sex anxiety, Oedipal rivalry and most probably male sex envy can be regarded as closely related though analytically separable components of a single emotional complex (Oedipal) that originates in a prolonged and intimate association between mother and son. But whereas mother-son intimacy may be considered a universal and perhaps even sufficient cause of male sex anxiety, the other two components of the complex are only likely to be of sufficient strength to seek overt expression in male ritual when the society is so structured that either the sexes or adjacent generations form sharply differentiated social groups or categories (1967:21).

According to this hypothesis the Bena Bena, like the Sambia and others, should display both male sex envy and Oedipal rivalry along with (universal?) male sex anxiety. This is so because there is a long postpartum sex taboo, sons sleep with their mothers, women are sharply differentiated from men and males are age graded. I contend, however, that in the case of the Bena Bena, Oedipal conflict as described by Spiro does not occur. Thus, as the Bena Bena have essentially the same initiation rites as other New Guinea Highlanders such as Gahuku-Gama, Fore, Auyana, Tairora, and others, and rites that are similar in some respects to those in other New Guinea societies, such rites can exist without the Oedipal component. I submit the following arguments which may or may not apply to other cases in the New Guinea Highlands or elsewhere.

First, let us accept Spiro's description of the Oedipus complex:

> The male Oedipus complex, according to Freud, basing his description on clinical evidence, is a *triangular* constellation involving a boy, his father, and his mother, in which the boy's *sexual desire* for the mother, whose love he wishes to monopolize, *leads* to hostility toward his father (and his siblings), whom he views as a rival for the mother's love. As a result of his wish to possess the exclusive love of the mother, the boy moreover develops the wish to kill the father and to replace him in his

relationship with the mother. (In the mind of a little boy, of course, "to kill" means to eliminate, to banish, to be rid of.)

> Love and hatred for his mother and father, respectively, are not the only feelings that the boy has for them. On the contrary, his feelings are highly ambivalent. Since typically the mother spurns the boy's erotic advances, her seeming preference for his rival, the husband-father, also evokes the boy's hostility toward her. Similarly, although the boy hates his father because he perceives him to be a rival for the love of the mother, he also loves and admires him for his protection and nurturance (1982:4).

Spiro is careful to point out that ". . . it is not that the boy hates his father *and* loves his mother, but rather that he hates his father *because* he loves his mother" (1982:4). He then goes on to explain that:

> The Oedipus complex is brought into being not by the boy's hatred of the father, but by his love—and specifically his sexual love—for the mother, his first "love-object." To be sure, the mother initially becomes his love-object not because of his sexual desire for her, but "as a result of her feeding him and looking after him" (Freud [1931] 1968:228). At this early ("oral") stage of psychosexual development, however, the boy's love for the mother is "pre-Oedipal"; his *Oedipal* love for her is associated with a later ("phallic") stage of psychosexual development, the stage at which—toward the end of the third year of life—the genitals achieve libidinal primacy. It is at this time that the boy's hostility to the father, whom he now perceives as his rival for the love of the mother, comes into being . . . (1982:5).

Psychoanalyst Robert J. Stoller, who has worked closely with Gilbert Herdt on the Sambia materials, regards the pre-Oedipal period as crucial because, he argues, "the Oedipal explanation, though correct, is incomplete" (1985:196). This general psychoanalytic perspective has also been the key element in John W. M. Whiting's explanations for the correlation between male initiation rites, long postpartum sex taboos, and exclusive mother-son sleeping arrangements (Whiting, Kluckhohn and Anthony 1958; Burton and J.W.M. Whiting 1961). There are two variations on the basic argument. In the first of the two, where fathers are absent for a time, there is a long postpartum sex taboo, and the boys sleep with and have an exceptionally close relationship with mother. Thus, they resent it when the father returns; the child feels replaced in the affection of his mother, identifies with mother and is hostile to father. In the second and later version the gist of the argument is that boys spend the first few years of life in intimate (or "exclusive") association with their mothers (which includes sleeping with them) and fathers are typically absent and/or aloof. Therefore the boys make a primary cross-sex identification and are in danger of being "feminized." They must undergo a "radical resocialization" at adolescence if they are to become fully "masculinized." In the case of the Sambia and some other New Guinea groups this involves male homosexuality although very similar rites can and do exist without this particular element (see Herdt 1981, 1982, 1987, Stoller 1985, 1985a, and Stoller and Herdt 1985, for the most detailed expositions of this view). The purpose of the rites, then, is to accomplish this resocialization, turn the boys into men and warriors, and to "contain" the Oedipal wishes of the boys while at the same time gratifying the "complementary Oedipal complex of the men" (Spiro 1982:170).

As the kinds of ethnographic details about marriage and childrearing necessary to demonstrate the accuracy of this view are largely absent for the New Guinea Highlands in particular and New Guinea in general, it is difficult to determine precisely what occurs during the childrearing process.[3] Thus these claims are little more than assumptions based upon ethnographic glosses which need more careful scrutiny than they have received to date. Let us begin with the notion of intimate or exclusive mother-son ties.

First, I remind you that clans in the New Guinea Highlands were relatively small autonomous groups seldom exceeding 250 persons. In the Bena Bena area, and most others, clan members rarely traveled far from their own territory. There

[3] But see Bambi Schieffelin's recent account of language socialization of Kaluli children (1990).

was strong solidarity and everyone was well known to everyone else. The birth of a child was known about and shared by all. All females in the clan old enough to be the child's mother could be called by that term and all other females could be termed sisters. The terms implied nurturance and in fact virtually all clanswomen were nurturant toward the infant even though, naturally, the actual mother of the child was usually dominant in this respect. Infants were nursed when they cried and, unlike the case for the Yandapu Enga (Gray 1982:83), could be nursed by females other than their mother. Infants could on rare occasions also be seen sucking on the dry breasts of grandmothers. Whether being suckled or not, infants and toddlers were commonly passed from person to person and received affection from all. They were generally weaned by the time they were approximately three. This same general pattern of childrearing occurs among the Fore (Sorenson 1976) and was so strong among the nearby Tairora that Watson was led to describe it in terms of "collective nurturance" (1983:265), in which the "nurturant collectivity is a generationally defined group of parents" (1983:271). He also describes this in terms of "the community-as-parent" (1983:273).[4]

While infants were still nursing they accompanied their mothers, usually sleeping in a net-bag suspended from the

---

4 Kurtz has written an interesting paper on the importance of Trobriand Islander's play groups in socializing children (1991). He criticizes both Malinowski and Spiro for not taking these important group factors into account with respect to helping the youngsters overcome their Oedipal feelings for their mothers. But see Spiro's reply (1992) and Kurtz's response (1993). Without going into detail I would argue that although Bena Bena play groups may well be important for socialization they are nothing like those of the Trobriand Islands with respect to the free sexual play that characterizes the latter.

Spiro has more recently been taken to task in an important and detailed paper by Patrick Glass who argues Trobriand ethnography needs to be more carefully examined, "in the light of important data on traditional beliefs and knowledge of paternity," which changes rather dramatically our view of the Trobriand family. He concludes that ". . . The Oedipus myth is not a universal paradigm to explain all family life and social organisation" (1996: from the abstract).

mother's forehead and hung on a nearby tree while the mother was working. As the women typically worked in groups there was usually more than one child to be cared for and there was also typically an older clan sister or a premenstrual bride in attendance for this purpose. When male infants became toddlers and nursed less frequently they did not always accompany their mothers. Boys and girls played together as toddlers but this changed quickly and by four or five they began to play almost exclusively with children of their own gender. Female children continued to accompany their mothers and were schooled in women's work and duties. Although male toddlers were usually supervised by an older female sibling, supervision even at this young age tended to be minimal and the boys ran and played pretty much as they chose. If they climbed too high or otherwise got into danger they would usually be rescued, but not until the situation was extremely dangerous by Western European standards. It was not at all unusual to see even very small toddlers playing with sharp bush knives with no intervention on the part of caretakers (see Sorenson 1976:168). Boys went entirely naked until approximately seven years of age; girls wore a small string apron virtually from birth.

While it was true that infants and toddlers slept with their mothers in the mothers' houses, how exclusive an arrangement this was (apart from the exclusion of adult males) is open to question. As there was no such thing as an only child (except, of course, firstborns) there were always siblings who shared the mother's bed (a raised platform which occupied roughly half of the small circular women's house). As children nursed less frequently and/or were weaned they tended to sleep together in the women's houses with their chums. Both men and women sometimes put an old net-bag over their head, blackened their teeth and frightened these groups of children. They thought this very funny. As people slept only when they were tired and did not seem to require silence, it was possible even in the middle of the night to hear both children and adults quietly talking and laughing.

A number of Bena Bena customs tended to promote multiple parenting and caretaking. For example, all little girls were "marked" by a clansman other than their father who became responsible for their initiation and subsequently received their bride-price. "Men," the Bena Bena said, "cannot take pay for their own semen." These relationships usually involved affection between the "adopting" family and the child. Similarly, the adoption of boys was relatively common in Bena Bena as well as elsewhere in New Guinea (Berndt 1962, Codrington 1969, Hallpike 1977, Held 1957, Lindenbaum 1979, Robbins 1982, Watson 1983). But the boys did not usually leave the clan, they simply changed the place where they typically slept and ate and thus in effect maintained multiple parents. Likewise, it was common for a man, if he took a particular fancy to a child, to create a special relationship with him (or her, occasionally) by giving the child his name. There was a special reciprocal term for this, *apatnigasi,* which resulted in bonds of genuine and lasting affection. As it was necessary to have daughters in order to provide wives for sons, it was my impression that these customs allowed people to balance their families in such a way as to insure these results. One consequence of this was the multiplication of personal ties between families and subclans and the further dilution of exclusive parental bonds. It was also not unusual for even small children to choose to spend the night or even a few days with their father's brother or some other clansman (Langness 1965, 1969, 1972, 1972a, 1974, 1975, 1981).

Bena Bena children, from the time they were infants, received a great deal of affection from clan mothers and sisters (and others as we shall see below). While it is true to say they slept and spent time with their mothers, their childrearing experiences when compared with Western European standards were quite different. Even as toddlers and youngsters they had a great deal of independence and played primarily in like-sexed groups. Although the mother-son bond was intimate, intimacy is a relative concept, and among the Bena Bena the relationship would not be well described as exclusive (also see Sorenson 1976). Indeed, women who had several children, who worked long hard hours daily, who ended their day coming in from their gardens with heavy loads of sweet potatoes and also carrying firewood, who then had to call and feed their pigs as well as cook the evening meal, would seem to have had little time to invest in giving exclusive attention to or infantilizing their sons. Ryder has made a similar observation for the Chimbu (1989). Furthermore, as women were well aware that their sons had to grow up to be warriors, and, indeed, took pride in the ritual advancement of their sons (Godelier 1986:153, Watson 1983:263), they had little incentive to do such things. Indeed, if you take the period from birth to age seven as salient, instead of merely the pre-Oedipal period, it could be argued that by Western European standards the boys were actually neglected by their mothers. Bena Bena boys after about age five were simply given a sweet potato in the morning and turned loose to do what they would.

It is claimed by Herdt and Stoller and apparently accepted by many that while in the (exclusive?) hands of women the little boys are "feminized." This is a poor choice of terms as the connotation in English is hard to overcome even when reminded that it is meant to apply to the feminine nature of New Guinea women. New Guinea women were not, in my opinion, very feminine in the English meaning of that term. This argument would seem to imply, among other things, that the boys were being taught feminine tasks. This was certainly not true in the Bena Bena case. They did not help women with their gardening, they were not taught women's gardening magic, they did not learn to make net-bags or string, they rarely if ever baby sat, they were taught nothing about childbirth or childcare nor, in fact, did they have or perform duties of any kind. As soon as they were physically able they basically just ran wild, getting into mischief, willfully doing whatever they pleased, and were rarely if ever punished. Mothers would sometimes yell and threaten their children but such threats fell upon deaf ears and usually failed to materialize.

This was not unique to the Bena Bena. It was true of the Ndumba and probably many other Melanesians as well: "The life of a Ndumba boy (*nraammwa*) is one of play and indulgence, with virtually no explicit discipline and no responsibilities (in contrast to a Ndumba girl, whose child-care and gardening tasks begin early in life)" (Hays 1987:188; also see Sorenson 1976). Apparently the situation is much the same for the Sambia: "Sambia children are rarely punished, for fear it will stunt their growth. Fathers, unlike mothers, do not reprimand their children, a fact that enters into the ordeals of submission expected from initiation" (Herdt and Stoller 1990:251). Bena Bena parents also virtually never punished their children as it was believed that until they were at least seven or so they were incapable of either understanding or reasoning. At worst the Bena Bena case might be said to be similar to the Trobriands: "People will sometimes grow angry with their children and beat them in an outburst of rage; but I have quite as often seen a child rush furiously at his parent and strike him. This attack might be received with a good-natured smile, or the blow might be angrily returned; but the idea of definite retribution, or of coercive punishment, is not only foreign, but distinctly repugnant to the native" (Malinowski 1929:45).

As Bena Bena women were aggressive in their dealings with other women, and also toward their husbands when angry, as they subscribed to the same values of "strength" and "hardness" as did men, and as they encouraged this in their children, it is difficult to see how they could be said to have been feminizing their sons. As Hays has suggested, "Boys are socialized to be *boys*" (1994). Some idea of the basic "flavor" of Bena Bena childrearing can be seen in the following excerpt from my fieldnotes:

"B and his wife, I, were sitting by the fire in front of I's house this evening. B gave a stick to F, his three-year-old son, with instructions to 'stick it up Y's vagina,' Y being his six-year-old daughter. F proceeded to try to do just that, chasing Y around the yard poking at her with the stick. Y started to cry. Both B and his wife laughed and apparently thought this to be very funny."

Sorenson has pointed out that among the Fore, "Aggressive acts by toddlers and young children was considered natural, and no attempt was made to chastise or punish them, nor was anger or marked displeasure usually shown" (1976:180). Similarly, aggression on the part of male children was valued among the Mae Enga of the Western Highlands: ". . . boys find time to scuffle and brawl among themselves, and their fathers are content to see them exhibit the aggressiveness that will be useful to them later" (Meggitt 1977:61). Newman (1989) reports that when Awa boys throw tantrums, which they do frequently, adults put sticks or clubs in their hands and direct them toward the source of their frustration.

Bena Bena boys sometimes beat their clan sisters (although at other times they could be terribly affectionate toward them) and openly boasted about having done so. Neither mothers or fathers punished them for this. When children fought, parents rarely intervened unless it continued too long. Neither men or women cried, except rarely, and, again like the Fore (Sorenson 1976), they paid little or no attention to children crying except in the case of hungry infants, who they immediately picked up and attempted to feed or otherwise mollify (see also B. Schieffelin 1990).

Women of the clan argued openly at times and fights between co-wives were by no means uncommon. These sometimes involved serious physical violence and even an occasional death as the women attacked each other with the rough planks that were used to fasten their doorways, tore at each other's clothing and hair, and wrestled each other to the ground. As role models they were hardly what Western Europeans would regard as either passive or feminine. Young girls fought aggressively also, even with sisters: "At home in the women's house and the cooking grove, however, the younger girl protests when her sister issues what seem to be arbitrary commands, and they fight savagely. The older girl may use brute force to beat the younger into submission" (Reay 1959:78). Men, in fact, valued these qualities in women, and would often comment admiringly that "so and so is a strong woman." When women fought, men seldom intervened, again, unless it continued for too long. A better idea of how far a "strong" woman could go can be seen in this somewhat unusual case from Auyana:

> At the opposite extreme was Pu'a, a quiet, tongue-tied, shy young man in his middle twenties in 1962. Pu'a had somehow been matched with a flirtatious, loud-mouthed, assertive woman. As their house was close to mine, I heard many arguments between them and the tongue lashings she gave him. The ultimate degradation arose when he decided to donate a pig which she did not want killed. Knowing she would attack him in order to prevent him from killing it, he told some men in his pooling unit that he wanted to donate the pig and for them to kill it. They cheerfully did so the morning of the pooling. Pu'a's wife did not interfere and did nothing except avoid him until he came home that evening after the distribution had been completed. As he entered the house, she screamed at him for having killed the pig and hurled vicious insults. He only shouted back at her occasionally. By this time, we all were intently listening in order not to miss any part of the show. Suddenly there was a howl and Pu'a staggered out of the door with his wife flailing at him with a firebrand. Just as he got outside, she smashed him on top of the head, knocking him to his knees. She took one brief look at him, whirled around, and stalked back into the house. He knelt a few seconds, appearing dazed and then got up and staggered back into the house. Nothing further was heard (Robbins 1982:87).

Similarly, among the Baktaman: "Warfare is also a male prerogative, in which women are expected to be the passive victims. . . . In domestic quarrels, on the other hand, the wife is often violent and beats her husband with firewood or other objects. Men do not feel dishonoured by such treatment, and freely complain of the resulting pains and bruises to arouse public sympathy" (Barth 1975:203).

Among the Melpa there can arise somewhat similar situations: "Thus in the not very usual case of an unequally matched pair, where the wife is the stronger partner and is seen to take a directive in their affairs, others may say that she is really the man, 'the woman has turned into a man', in relation to her husband" (M. Strathern 1978:189). Indeed, according to Marilyn Strathern, among the Melpa "It is an insult for a woman to be singled out as exemplifying feminine traits, as it is praise for a man to be called a man" (1978:188). Berndt, writing about Eastern Highlanders, says: "Women, too, are taught as they grow to adulthood that it is good to fight, to be strong, and to assert themselves" (1962:402). Van Baal says of Marind-anim women: ". . . Of course, the Marind-anim woman is not so easily made the victim of male cruelty. She is perfectly capable of defending herself both with a sharp tongue and with a pair of sturdy hands" (1966:168).

When a Bena Bena woman refused to accept an arranged marriage and ran away to a different place, most probably to a former lover, her father, guardian, and brothers would find her and bring her back, sometimes rather brutally. But if she was persistent and kept running away there was no recourse for them but to give in to her wishes and return the bride-price. They would say of her, with begrudging admiration, "She is strong. We can't make her stay." Similarly, among the Melpa: "If a woman is adamant for divorce, she gets her way. 'It is her own strength of will,' men say" (Strathern and Strathern 1969:153). Pospisil says of Kapauku: ". . . when a girl is determined, no one can force her into any marriage" (1964:53).

While it was the case that uninitiated Bena Bena boys were regarded as polluting because of their contacts with women, this was apparently a much milder version of that belief than that found among either Sambia (Herdt 1981) or Hua (Meigs 1984). Similarly, while it was also the case that at least in infancy they might be said to have inhabited primarily a "women's world," to say they were regarded as feminine because of this would be to truly stretch the point. Indeed, to claim there was a "woman's world" (Weiner 1976) of any great significance in the Eastern Highlands would probably be to stretch the point. In this sense the Bena Bena were much like the Marind-anim about whom Van Baal made what might well be seen as a classic of male chauvinism: "The inadequacy of the relations between the sexes is sustained by another peculiar facet of Marind-anim culture. It is a culture of males and the women have no culture of their own" (1966: 952). Although extreme, I do not believe this is far from the truth.

While there were, of course, certain things done exclusively by women, to talk of a significant female culture as opposed to a male or Bena Bena culture in general would be, again, an exaggeration. Even though women did not attain them to the same degree, men and women shared the basic values of the culture, which I would take to be generosity, independence, strength, and competence. Faithorn has made much the same point with respect to the nearby Kafe (1976) as has Marilyn Strathern for the Melpa:

> In no sense do Hagen women have a sub-culture of their own analogous to men's. In terms of ritual, ceremony, song and such like, there is very little female specialisation. The specialisation must rest in areas as yet undiscovered. On the surface, women's alternative value-system would seem to consist almost entirely of resistance, of assertions of autonomy in particular situations (e.g. the role of wife) regarded by men as non-ideal even if typical. Yet the idea of non-conformism has not been developed to the point of an ideology or tradition, though one might in behavioral terms look for a "sub-culture" here. Assertions of autonomy are not of course restricted to females. In a way, this is another example of women making use of notions shared also by men (1978:184).

The situation among the Hua is similar: "Conversely, women, through their consumption of food associated with the *hakeri'a* qualities of men, attempt to achieve some male characteristics. At menstruation, after childbirth, and in efforts at contraception, women eat small bits of *hakeri'a* leaves. The one most commonly used is brown, dried out, and extremely hard. The women's stated intention is to induce a dryness and hardness in the womb so that the menstrual or postparturitional flow will be reduced and fertility inhibited. Women who achieve such a condition of the womb, according to the Hua, neither menstruate nor conceive. Such women proudly claim to be like men" (Meigs 1984:61–62). Van Baal says of the Marind-anim: "The facts are that they [Marind-anim women] adopted male ideals and culture-patterns as their own. They glorified in male activities and male beauty as exhibited in dance and ritual. They did their utmost to make their own men into brightly-coloured birds of paradise, contenting themselves with the same modest and inconspicuous feathers as the female bird" (Van Baal 1966:170).

This brings up a further point that needs clarification, the distinction between being male and female and being masculine and feminine. Aside from the case of hermaphrodites (which I never encountered or even heard of in the Bena Bena) there was no doubt about an infant's sex. Boys possessed a penis and little girls did not. As in Auyana: "The criterion of sex was binary, agreed upon at birth, and was nonnegotiable. Strong women might act like men and weak men might act like women but for a person to become the opposite sex was only a fantasy . . ." (Robbins 1982:163). That Bena Bena boys were male was known to everyone as they went naked until approximately age seven and little girls did not. This identification was made even more apparent by the fact that people commented about the little boys' penes, frequently pulled on or fondled them, and thus constantly called special attention to them. Men, it was true, quite commonly threatened to cut them off, but as this was so common and so obviously done in jest it seems not to have bothered the boys very much. For example, on one occasion I witnessed an adult clansman tell a boy of about four that he would cut off his penis. The boy looked at him for a couple of seconds and then calmly replied, "you have a big nose." Everyone laughed. On another occasion I saw a women playfully threaten her son (of about six) that she would bite his penis off. There was a great deal of fondling of the boy's penes by males. Women fondled infants but not older boys. Individuals of both sexes would pick up infants and mouth their genitals and kiss them all over.[5] There was an enormous amount of physical contact between clanpersons of all kinds, except husbands and wives. While this did have a sensual quality to it, it is important to remember that it occured in a culture where the traditional greeting meant, "I eat your genitals," and one in which every part of a person was believed to be an important element in their very being—hair, urine, feces, fingernails, pus, phlegm, and certainly the skin. In addition to the verbal greeting, men (and women, too) would embrace each other, touch each other's genitals, and rub their hands all over the other person's body often for several minutes at a time. To interpret all this fondling as simply "sexual" must be carefully considered. In this respect the Bena Bena were similar to their neighbors, the Gahuku-Gama (Read 1952, 1954, 1955, 1965), the Fore (Sorenson 1976), and probably to most other Eastern Highlanders. I would take exception to Marilyn Strathern's recent interpretive *tour de force* in which she argues that male and female are not fixed points but, rather, exist only as they situationally reveal themselves out of androgynous forms (1988:184). For the Bena Bena at least, as far as I can determine, they are fixed. This does not mean that males cannot behave in what they perceive as female ways and vice versa, but the idea of an androgynous creature I think would be

5 This is widespread in Papua New Guinea. Gillison writes of the Gimi: "Masturbation is another pacifying technique. With a baby girl, the mother or *amau* holds her hand over the vulva and shakes it vigorously. She may kiss the vagina, working her way up the middle of the body to the lips and then inserting her nipple (often when the child has given no sign of discontent). With a boy, she kisses the penis, pulls at it with her fingers and takes it into her mouth to induce an erection. Several women may pass a baby boy back and forth, each one holding him over her head as she takes a turn sucking or holding the penis in her mouth. When the child then pulls at his own organ, the women, greatly amused, offer squeezes and pulls of their own" (1993:176). Only the genitals of males are fondled by the Gururumba (Newman 1962:167). Somewhat similar behaviors have been reported for other Highlands groups as well (Berndt 1962:91–92; Brandewie 1981:65; Hogbin 1943:298).

lost on them.[6] Along these lines it might be pointed out that there are no "berdache" in New Guinea.[7]

Male toddlers were given miniature bamboo bows and arrows by their fathers and encouraged to practice. Girls were not supposed to touch bows and arrows (although they sometimes did). Boys were present when pigs are being butchered and, indeed, were often underfoot and roughly shoved aside. Girls were much less present at such male tasks and then mainly on the sidelines. Boys, as in the case quoted above, were actively encouraged to dominate girls. Even when young, long before they were to be initiated, they were encouraged by men and their peers not to spend time with their mothers. They were, in fact, treated differently in virtually every way. Thus, granted that being male was not identical with being masculine (or perhaps more appropriately, "manly") as Herdt and Stoller argue, there could be no doubt in anyone's mind that Bena Bena boys were male and not female, and there must have been at least some significance in a boy's early recognition of this simple and basic fact.[8] This is especially true in that as far as I know the Bena Bena, apparently like the Sambia (Herdt, 1981:168), did not themselves distinguish sex from gender. Thus masculine (male) gender (sexual?) identification began very early and was continuous: it did not just settle itself during male initiation rites as Herdt and Stoller seem to imply for the Sambia. It is interesting that when discussing a Sambia deviant they comment that when he faced the initiation he wished he had been born a girl, "a desire

---

6 Marilyn Strathern does not argue that Melanesians in fact think in this way. She says of this, ". . . I have not presented Melanesian ideas but an analysis from the point of view of Western anthropological and feminist preoccupations of what Melanesian ideas might look like if they were to appear in the form of those preoccupations" (1988:309). In spite of this disclaimer James F. Weiner seems to accept the idea of androgynous forms as real in his analyses of Papua New Guinea myths (1995).

7 However, Gray (1982) reports one Yandapu Enga man with gynecomastia (enlarged breasts) who considered himself a woman, dressed and worked as one, and was married to a man who also had other wives. Unfortunately no other details are reported.

8 See B. Schieffelin (1990) for a fairly detailed account of gender socialization among the Kaluli.

unheard of from Sambia men" (Herdt and Stoller 1990:283). B. Schieffelin says of Kaluli: "Kaluli mothers socialize their sons into masculine roles from the very beginning of their devlopment. My data show that for the first three to four years of a child's life, Kaluli mothers are the major caregivers. In their interactions with their sons, they teach them gender-appropriate behavior, just as they teach their daughters appropriate ways to act" 1990:205).

Why, in these cultures, given women's relative low status and powerlessness, would a male child identify or overidentify with his mother? Further, what can it mean to claim that male children inhabited a "female world" (Read 1982, Herdt 1981) when, although in primary association with female caretakers during infancy, those caretakers were not in important respects "feminine," did not instruct them in female ways, and, indeed, encouraged them to acquire the presumably "male values" of strength and aggressiveness? The Bena Bena case is very unlike the Baruya case, for example, where, according to Godelier: "Till then [age seven], he lives in the world of women, dressed in a long *pulpul* similar to the skirts worn by little girls. Indeed, he plays with his sisters, female cousins, and female neighbors" (1986:31). I assume Godelier means that he "also" plays with sisters and so forth. Similarly, given the Eastern Highlander's beliefs about females in general, and the female genitals in particular,[9] why would one expect to find "womb envy?" (Lidz and Lidz 1989). I will return to this issue later.

And what of absent and/or aloof fathers? It is not my experience that Bena Bena fathers were absent either physically or psychologically although it is certainly true they slept in

[9] In some parts of New Guinea the female genitals are regarded as so frightening that exposing them is believed to frighten off malevolent beings. ". . . Suddenly the women all pulled aside their pubic coverings and flashed their vulvas at him. Hides was quite taken aback and mystified at this surprising act. He did not know they were treating him as a malevolent supernatural being and were trying to defuse his power and chase him away" (Schieffelin and Crittenden 1991:140).

the men's houses and, in important respects, avoided contact with females. Typically a man visited his wife and children at his wife's house for a late afternoon meal. If he had more than one wife, as approximately 25 percent of the Bena Bena males where I worked did, he took turns visiting them. One of the first signs of marital strife or pending divorce was a man's failure to do this. He accepted sweet potatoes cooked by his wife for himself and his children and usually ate his meal in their company. He carried away cooked sweet potatoes for his breakfast and/or lunch the next day. The children did likewise.

Far from being aloof, Bena Bena fathers were affectionate and even demonstrative with their children of both sexes, holding them, cuddling them, giving them little gifts of pork, and so forth. A man could not see his infant child for the first month (again, a very moderate version of a widespread Highlands avoidance pattern) and, while it was true there was a taboo against a man carrying his first born child, men had more than one child and they also had adopted children and others to carry if they wished. Similarly, as among Hua, these taboos appeared to be more serious at the verbal level than the behavioral: ". . . A man may not carry his firstborn baby (male or female) on his shoulders lest he be prematurely 'put or pressed down.' Nonetheless the Hua are warm, loving, and gentle with their children: resentment of the firstborn is expressed verbally and symbolically, never to my knowledge physically" (Meigs 1984:104). Bena Bena men would sometimes take their sons with them while they were making or repairing garden fences, building houses, digging garden ditches, or engaging in other domestic activities. They were proud of their children and did not hide their feelings about them, especially when they were "strong" and handsome (when they had clear, lighter skins, aquiline noses, and were tall and physically adept). Because the gardens of the Bena Bena who inhabit the grasslands immediately surrounded the villages rather than being more distant, the adult males were usually working nearby where they could be seen by everyone including children.

Similarly, because hunting is virtually absent among the grassland-dwelling Bena Bena, men were rarely away from their own villages and even then only for days rather than weeks as in the case of the Baruya or Sambia (Godelier 1986:14; Herdt 1981:138). Public events at which fathers presided were frequent and witnessed by everyone including children. Cooking with earth ovens, for example, a common event in Bena Bena life, was always done by men and witnessed by everyone. Men were an everyday presence in village life just as were women. Thus while they may have been absent from the mother's house during the night they were not often absent from the village or from the "life space" of their children. Some quotes from my field notes illustrate this:

"March 22, 1961: Even very small children spend quite a lot of time with their fathers. You can often see the men sitting around holding a child. Sometimes when a child is tired he will be held until he falls asleep and then put down somewhere. The children, of course, run to their fathers for protection. When I come around, for example, if they are afraid they will run to their fathers who invariably hold them until they are ready to run off and play again."

"April 21, 1961: Fimaso (about 2) cried today when Bonobo (his father) tried to leave him with his mother. Finally the parents gave in (as usual) and Fimaso ran down the path after Bonobo. . . .

"Children are spoiled very badly by the men—less so, but also, by the women. But in any case they are rarely disciplined, seldom punished, and usually get their way. They do little work to speak of but do sometimes carry firewood, food, or *pit pit* (cane). Also an older boy will sometimes sleep in the gardens to chase pigs away."

"April 26, 1961: The men treat all the boys more or less like their own sons. Today, for example, Abio was walking with his son Finamuna (about 4). Amuloya, Sepik's boy (about

5) came up and began talking to Abio and held his hand. Later, in Sapuro village, Abio called out to Finamuna to go with him to his coffee. Finamuna was playing and did not heed so he and Amuloya walked off hand in hand. . . .

"Today Tubutaboe gave some pig fat to Mate (about 3), a girl whom he has 'marked.' Cilarki tried to give her a piece also but she just made a face at him and refused it. Tubutaboe then took it from Cilarki and held it out to her and she accepted it. A man who has marked a girl like this seems to go out of his way to be nice to her. . . .

"Even small children of 3 or 4 wander about by themselves, gathering passion fruit, playing and so on. No one seems to worry about them. Often I will see Yosimi or Gooyi (both about 3 or 4) or other children about that size playing either in the village or in a garden with no older person in sight. This is by no means uncommon."

"May 13, 1961: The boys seem to resent it if a boy walks around with his mother rather than his age mates. Today Bianiso (about 7) remarked about one boy that he didn't pal around with them but went all the time with his mother. All of the boys expressed their disapproval of his behavior."

"June 23, 1961: Vissise was smoking and Gemlepa (his son of about 5) walked up to him and said, 'your skin is on fire.' He took Vissise's cigarette and put it out. Vissise did nothing. Gemlepa is constantly hanging around and onto Vissise and seems to genuinely worship him."

"July 20, 1961: The people, men especially, are much more tolerant of children than we (Europeans) are. A man will put up with any kind of climbing, pulling, pestering, etc. on the part of his children. When not moving about working or otherwise busy a man is almost constantly holding, petting, or talking to a child. Most frequently this is a boy but often girls as well."

"August 21, 1961: Bonanihi's wife was holding Wapio, Ietopesso's infant son. She remarked to a woman near her about the baby's genitals and then she took her hand and pretended to carry them to her mouth and eat them. She would touch them with her fingers and then put her fingers to her mouth as if kissing them. Later, Sepik's first wife was holding Wapio, kissing him on the stomach and holding him up and tickling his feet with her mouth, etc. Naguropave (a teenager) later came and took him from Ietopesso, also fondling him for a time."

"November 15, 1961: Men as well as women are extremely playful and affectionate with babies. This morning Sepik (an adult male) was holding Wapio (his adopted brother's infant son), flicking out his tongue at him and even in his mouth, talking 'baby talk' to him and so on. Wapio loved it. Kikipe (an older adult male of the subclan) held him also and made much of him. When Wapio looked as if he might cry Kikipe kidded him and sort of 'loved' him out of it. . . . Wareka is taking care of his baby today, holding it and fondling it. . . . The men make it a point to give food to the boys (and girls) when they are around. For example, while sitting there today waiting for the stones to heat, Afooya came with Finamuna (about 4) and his other little grandson (about the same age). Bonobo (an adult male) immediately broke off part of his tapioc and gave it to Finamuna. Klehopave (also an adult male) gave a piece of sweet potato to the other child and the two children were then encouraged by all the men present to eat it."

"March 31, 1962: Kaesso (an adult male) today, as Kano (about 3) passed by him, reached out and pulled on his penis. He then took the boy in his arms and fondled him. Later I saw Gugupa (an adult male) kissing a small boy.

"There is a great deal of affection between adults and children—and this has little to do with the family or subclan. Any adult is apt to love and fondle any child almost at random. Today, for example, I saw Kaesso (an adult male) fondling Kano (not of the same subclan), Gugupa (an adult male) kissing him, Bonanihi (an older adult male) fondling Mate (a girl of 3), Mumugefa (an older adult male) fondling her and Bubisso (a boy of about 5). Adults are very fond of children and very permissive and loving. Even so, today when all the men were gathered and three small boys were with them, when a small girl (about 8) came too close and peered over the fence Katopi (an adult male) got up with a switch and chased her away."

I could give many more similar examples. Prior to pacification, of course, fathers could not have had as much time as they did when my observations were made. It is also true that men were cautioned about spending too much time around children as well as around women. But I do not believe the basic pattern was different. They were not *always* at war. When groups were strong and dominant, as was the group of Bena Bena I worked with, there were substantial periods of time when life was relatively easy, gardens flourished, the pig herds could be increased to make possible the periodic exchanges (and initiations), and *people could enjoy their children.* I certainly do not believe that prior to pacification Bena Bena men were indifferent to their children, absent and aloof, and only learned to be affectionate and caring during the post-contact period. The Bena Bena may be different than other Highlanders in this respect, which I doubt, but to simply dismiss fathers and husbands as aloof or physically and psychologically absent is just not satisfactory. Fathers and husbands are far more absent from the ethnographic literature (indeed, they are amazingly absent from it) than they probably were from their families. The Bena Bena case is somewhat like that of the Siane described earlier by Salisbury:

> . . . After a relatively short period when young children are looked after exclusively by their mother, and when they visit their father for fondling and affection, the training of children is undertaken by males and females generally, rather than by the elementary families. As soon as boys are old enough to talk and to understand, they are toilet trained by their fathers and by older boys: after their ceremonial weaning between the ages of 3 and 6, their principal companions are other boys (1962:18).

The Bena Bena case also seems to be somewhat similar to

that of the Gadsup:

> Parents, both the mother and to an increasing degree, as the child matures, also the father, play with the infant, tickling him while making gutteral sounds in simulation of those the infant makes. At about this time, the father may spend a few hours with the infant on his lap while the mother is away in the garden, visiting her relatives in some neighboring village, or attending a ceremony in her natal village. His treatment of the infant resembles closely that of the mother. Such motives as personal contact and reaction to the slightest sound from the infant characterizes his reactions. He constantly touches, strokes and pats the child. He may be relieved by a female sibling or daughter, but on the other hand he may spend a whole morning caring for the infant (Du Toit 1975:215).

Indeed, according to Reay, it was the father's greater nurturance that helped the boys begin to identify with their agnatic descent group: "A 'big' boy learns from his mother about the informal power women sometimes exercise. He can successfully evade compliance with his father's commands, but if he neglects the tasks (to provide kindling and drinking water) set by his mother, she can and does refuse to give him food. . . . The contrast between a permissive father and a mother who may starve him to induce conformity encourages a boy's identification with the agnatic descent group" (1959:169). Read described the basic pattern in *The High Valley* very succinctly: ". . . although they [children] often appeared to be neglected, they were showered with demonstrative affection" (1965:172).[10] In the Waina-Sowanda area fathers fondle and play with their children at around one year of age and the father's role in socialization between ages three and eight is said to be of crucial significance (Gell 1975:95).

[10]Kenneth Read unfortunately has never provided an account of Gahuku childrearing and is somewhat inconsistent on this point. In another publication he says, "Gahuku men had very little to do with boys until they were ten or a little older. After their birth, they were almost exclusively nurtured by women; men, including their older brothers, belonged to a different and in some sense physically separated world—a menacing world into whose perimeters they were wrenched for the first time at their early ritual washing" (1982:70). This is very unlike the Bena Bena case even though some Bena Bena married into Gahuku groups. It would be useful to know what "very little" actually means. Certain passages in *The High Valley* indicate to me that fathers certainly did at times interact with their small children.

Among the Baktaman:

> A newborn child is tended continuously by its mother until she resumes gardening, usually after one to two months. For a while it may be carried to the gardens and continue with its mother. As soon as convenient it is given to a *menkwap* "child tender." Such a person is usually an older child, and a person will always know who was its "child tender." This relationship obtains only among members of the same family or domestic unit, including stepchildren and foster children. A first child may have only its father as "child tender" (Barth and Reitan 1980:284).

Among the Abelam: ". . . To the mother falls much of the care of the child during infancy; it is fed frequently, caressed and fondled. When she is working, it is placed in a strong net-bag, and hung up on the fence or a tree in the shade. The father sees less of the child, but he pets it, and often carries it up to the piazza, where he sits talking with the other men. Sometimes he helps to feed it with taro or yam soup, revealing infinite patience in his attempts to make the child eat" (Kaberry 1941:246).

These cases appear to be quite different from the pattern of the Bimin-Kuskusmin farther to the west where it is said that boys for the first time have "close physical and affectionate contact with their fathers in public" only *after* initiation (Poole 1982:133).[11]

Although it is difficult to tell, in spite of Herdt's unusually detailed ethnography, it would appear that Sambia males may not be entirely different from Bena Bena in their treatment of their sons, the difference perhaps being only in the relative ages at which men significantly interact with them. Herdt reports that "Exceptionally close maternal attachment, prolonged orality, and physical and psychological distance from one's father are, therefore, key factors in early Sambia socialization." However, in the next paragraph he says, "In spite of this deliberately distanced beginning, most men are affectionate toward their older children, and they take a special pride in their sons." Earlier on the same page he says, "Both boys

[11]One might well wonder what transpires between father and child in private.

and girls sleep with their fathers occasionally. . . . For a year or two after weaning this is permitted; but the older a boy is, the more uncomfortable men become" (1981:214). On the following page he says, "Men let their wives and women rear their sons. But at three and four and five years of age there is a change: a father should begin to spend more time with his son. He should teach, direct, and push him, funneling his experiences in ways that separate mother and son and masculinize the boy" (1981:215). Elsewhere he speaks of paternal love: "This initiation combines the care of paternal love and the bite of cold-hearted military education" (1981:53).

It is my impression that Sambia may differ in their attitudes and treatment of their sons only in that perhaps there is less contact between fathers and sons when the latter are infants. With respect to caretaking the two cultures appear at least superficially to be similar: ". . . All adults tend to become caretakers and authorities over children." (Herdt, 1981:34) But even if Herdt is absolutely correct in his emphasis on the exclusiveness of the mother-son dyad, in order to accept his interpretation of Sambia rites one must believe that core identity is not only "fairly well formed by a year and half or two years" (Stoller 1973:314) but that it must be virtually irreversible by that time, because if it is "almost irreversible by around age five or six" (Stoller 1973:314, quoted in Herdt 1982:83), the childrearing practices as described by Herdt would not produce the necessary "feminizing" effect on gender development. Furthermore, one would have to assume that the years between five and ten (and even beyond that) are largely irrelevant to identity formation, which seems highly unlikely. Similarly, as according to Spiro genuine Oedipal love begins at about age three, precisely the age at which the nurturant Sambia fathers come into prominence in the child's life, might we not expect this to impact importantly on the Oedipal constellation? Herdt essentially dismisses this issue on the grounds that more data are needed while at the same time emphasizing the pre-Oedipal period: "My own review of the New Guinea literature (1981:303–325) indicates, however, that pre-Oedipal development seems as basic and pervasive as the status-envy and post-Oedipal conflict factors postulated by Whiting and his colleagues" (1982:83).

In a later publication Herdt has modified his argument somewhat and now suggests that it is not absent fathers that are important in bringing about ritual homosexuality (and initiation rites?) but, rather, fathers who are present but unpredictably so, as this results in an ambivalent relationship between fathers and sons:

> The father's relationship to his children is best termed ambivalent . . . with the intensity of ambivalence a function of physical closeness in early development. Here ambivalence means that a boy is faced with contradictory ideas and feelings that produce conflictual fantasies and action. Though father is present soon after birth, mother is the stronger attachment figure, and father remains aloof from the child until later. The father's culturally conditioned aloofness is mediated by the degrees of sexual antagonism in the society . . . such that the greater the sexual polarity, the greater paternal aloofness, which the child experiences as ambivalent. Father's inconsistent daytime presence, and uncontrollable movements to the men's house and "off-limit" arenas, are problematic for the boy. Hence postpartum taboos, culturally mandated avoidance, sexual antagonism, and interpersonal hostility combine to form the basic psychological *conditions* of father's ambivalent bond to the child (1989:351).

This position is not inconsistent with the Bena Bena case but, again, requires much further detail with respect to just what fathers do vis-à-vis children. This is especially so given that ambivalence toward fathers is expected in all cases according to the Oedipal hypothesis. If Sambia males truly suffer from problems of gender identify it could be argued that it is a *result* of their homosexual practices rather than a *cause* of them. Thus I am very skeptical that "Masculinity is thus a product of a regime of ritualized homosexuality leading into manhood" (Herdt 1981:3).[12] The overwhelming emphasis on

[12]This is also inconsistent with Stoller's insistence that ". . . the core of one's gender

the importance of the first five years of socialization does not lend itself to this possibility. The Bedamini, who also engage in homosexual rites similar to those of the Sambia, appear to allow a great deal of individual variation with respect to socialization:

> From about two years upwards boys will spend more of their time with males and ultimately start sleeping in the men's dormitory. The exact age at which boys leave the women's rooms varies according to factors of individual personality or the death of mother or father, but most have done so at the age of five or six years. In daily activities boys may join women as well as men until about the age of ten years. Thus the transfer from a predominantly female to a male sphere of influence is gradual, quite informal, and individually variable (Sorum 1982:57).

The Bena Bena share most of the beliefs about women and men that are reported from all over Melanesia. They engaged in many of the same kinds of rituals. Bena Bena male initiations involved ear and nose piercing, bloodletting from tongue, nose, and urethra, cane swallowing, and vomiting. They also involved the use of semen although there was no homosexuality as far as I could determine. Women were believed to be polluting, primarily because of menstruation. They were said to be, and appeared to agree, that they were weak and inferior to men in every way. Men (and even boys) were actively discouraged from spending time with them. There were no overt displays of affection between husbands and wives (although there was a great deal of this between clan brothers and sisters). Sexual intercourse was engaged in privately and to produce offspring and, supposedly, not otherwise. After intercourse, aboriginally, men were expected to cleanse themselves by swallowing canes and nose bleeding themselves before returning to the men's house. I have been told that most men did so. If a man did not perform these actions he was

---

identity—the sense of being a male or a female—is laid down by the first three years of life and is pretty much unalterable thereafter. . . . If one has developed that sense unequivocally, later experiences can threaten it, forcing modifications upon one as one attempts to protect that core, but the core will remain" (Stoller 1975:73).

criticized by other men as he was polluting to them.

There were many taboos having to do with male/female relationships. Women could not touch men's hair, could not be above them in any way, could not cast their shadows on them, had to retire to their menstrual huts during their menses, could not garden or cook food for anyone at such times, and so on. Men worked together in groups as did women although sometimes a man and a woman would work together temporarily in an established garden. There were clearly male and female tasks. Women grew sweet potatoes and most introduced vegetables; men grew yams, bananas, and taro. Men fenced garden plots, mended fences, and dug drainage ditches after women had broken the ground with shovels. Men staked the labor intensive wing-bean gardens, women possessed the magic to make the beans grow. Women manufactured string, net-bags, and armbands, men made bows and arrows and ale decorations for the various events they were in charge of organizing. Girls almost exclusively fetched water in the long bamboo tubes they used for that purpose, although if no girl was present men and boys would do so. It was not that women were domestic and men were not but, rather, that men were engaged in and visible in both domestic and public endeavors and women much less so in the latter. I agree with Marilyn Strathern here, however, in so far as she argues that the greater female presence in domesticity does not denigrate women as social persons (1988:89).

Most Bena Bena beliefs about men and women, as well as the day-to-day behavior that reflects them, were not, indeed, could not have been entirely secret. Children growing up heard women being disparaged, they witnessed the care with which men approached females, they saw that men were in charge of public events and most everything else, that they ordered women about and in general dominated them. Although their parents did not actually reside together, husbands and wives each had their own space in the women's houses where they kept their sparse belongings. Children were aware of this from an early age. Thus, although nuclear families could be recognized, they existed in a special cultural context. When fathers interacted with their children they were almost totally nurturant. When they were absent they were known to be residing in the mysterious and prestigious men's house with other men and engaging in men's activities which were thought by everyone to be superior in every way. Thus, given multiple caretaking, the nurturant role of Bena fathers, the existence of the men's house, strong proscriptions relating to relations between husbands and wives, the absence of overt expressions of affection between husbands and wives, and given the beliefs about female pollution and the status of women in general, the privacy (and presumed infrequency) of the parental sex act, it is difficult for me to believe that fathers could be perceived to be rivals for mothers' attention, particularly sexual attention. It is equally difficult to understand why a child would envy his mother's status, and in this context it is also difficult to understand why a child's love of his mother would result in his hating his father. The entire ethos of Bena Bena culture worked against such an outcome.

There is a question here, of course, as to precisely what the mother's role might have been in bringing about Oedipal conflict. That is, it has been suggested by Whiting and others (Whiting, Kluckhohn, and Anthony 1958), that because of the long postpartum sex taboo women might well have been seeking sexual gratification from their sons. The question of New Guinea Highlanders heterosexual relationships is complex and paradoxical. It could be argued on the one hand that women, like men, must have greatly feared sex, but on the other that they, like Tairora men, "regard(ed) sexual intercourse as one of the most urgent and unremitting pleasures of life" (Watson 1983:101). It was not my impression that Bena Bena women were particularly seductive toward their sons (or, indeed, that they would have reason to be).

It could also be argued, of course, as Spiro suggests, that fathers were dealing with their own Oedipal problems during the violent initiations. It is quite clear from the literature as well as from my own fieldwork that the initiates' fathers were not themselves responsible for inflicting any of the brutality or pain (Godelier 1986, Robbins 1982:95). And among the Sambia, as well as the Bena Bena, they apparently took pains to control what happened to their sons: ". . . a man would be foolish to risk cruel ritual treatment toward his son in initiation at an alien dance ground where he lacked the presence of reliable supporters" (Herdt 1981:32). Similarly, among the Ndumba it is the fathers and their clansmen who attempt to hinder the initiation procession:

> To the outside observer, the boys could hardly hold their fathers and clan-mates responsible for this suffering and betrayal. Not only were they not the principal initiators, but they have been part of the group apparently trying to prevent the initiation from taking place. Thus, if the *'ummanra* ceremony produces feelings of betrayal, resentment, or hostility on the part of the initiates, surely it is more likely that these would be directed at their matrilateral, rather than patrilateral, kinsmen. . . . (Hays 1987:197).

Also, among Kuma, ". . . Each man is associated with a particular boy—his son, his younger brother, or a boy of his subclan who has no closer relatives. He protects the boy from undue harshness, and may even prevent him from participating in the more ardous rituals" (Reay 1959:173). In Auyana the initiates are "beaten with branches and clublike succulents by all the initiated male members of their pooling unit except their fathers and brothers" (Robbins 1982:95).[13] Among the Fore and others the rites are modified to accomodate youths felt not up to them:

> There is, too, recognition that not all boys or youths can participate fully (that is, some are not physically able or so inclined) in certain of the rites, and not all will be fitted for

[13] In fairness to those who subscribe to the Oedipal hypothesis Robbins also says, "It was said that the reason those from the boy's mother's natal pooling unit mutilated him rather than those from his own pooling unit was that the former went easy on him, whereas the latter might have killed him (1982:95).

> active fighting. For example, in the case of cane-swallowing, novices who express great fear are merely marked symbolically with the cane on chest and belly. In certain cases the severity of nose-bleeding, tongue-cutting, and penis-bleeding is also relaxed, depending on the attitude of the novice. This is not just a result of indirect alien contact, for it is apparent too in the Busarasa-Moke districts where indigenous features of initiation have been virtually unaffected (Berndt 1962:109).

Baktaman fathers, elder brothers, and uncles console the initiates "if some break down too badly" (Barth 1975:51). It must also be emphasized that during the initiations, at least among the Gahuku-Gama and Bena Bena, the adult male participants inflict the same pain upon themselves as upon the initiates, a fact difficult to reconcile with an Oedipal hypothesis: ". . . the boys are compelled to watch and assist the older men as they demonstrate the rites of vomiting and blood-letting. They are forced to hold the ends of the u-shaped lengths of cane which their seniors have thrust down their own throats, and to move these up and down while the latter retch in the water. Later, when their own turn comes, the men exhort them with the words: 'You have done this to us; now we do it to you'" (Read 1952:13).[14]

Without father-son rivalry no Oedipal complex could develop whatever the pre-Oedipal situation might have been. Thus, while Oedipal conflict *can be* postulated as an intervening variable in the ongoing drama of the Bena Bena, to use that concept in spite of what appears to be evidence to the contrary violates the law of parsimony (Occam's razor). While it may have been possible for some particular Bena Bena individual or family to experience Oedipal conflict, this cannot have been typical of the culture. Thus, if my argument has merit, the existence and persistence of male initiation rites among the Bena Bena must, and I believe can be explained without recourse to Oedipal considerations.

---

[14] Graber's attempt to put forth "A Psychocultural Theory of Male Genital Mutilation" (1981), following Reik (1975), would also appear to be without foundation if fathers do not initiate their sons.

Although Herdt and Stoller emphasize the importance of the pre-Oedipal period they do not neglect the Oedipal period itself (Stoller and Herdt 1985). And there are reasons to suppose that the classical Oedipal situation would indeed be more likely to occur in Sambia than in Bena Bena. For example, the Sambia pattern of father, mother, and children inhabiting a single hut (Herdt 1982:52) is totally unlike the men's house pattern of the Bena Bena and, indeed, most of the New Guinea Highlands. In this situation the nuclear family would appear to be a more identifiable and behavioral entity. And, if Sambia values pit men against women even more strongly in Sambia than elsewhere (1982:53), this, too, might exacerbate the situation. There is also perhaps a more "luxuriant" relationship between sons and their mothers than that which obtains in the Bena Bena (1982:72). It is entirely possible that, for whatever reasons, fathers' attitudes toward their sons truly are much more aloof and psychologically distant than that of Bena fathers and that, similarly, mothers' attitudes are much more nurturant. And, finally, there are ecological differences that may well be related to all this. Sambia gardens are further from the villages, necessitating more time away from the village. Hunting, which is virtually nonexistant in the grasslands of Bena Bena, also takes men away for long periods of time.

Whatever the result of Sambia childrearing practices, I find it virtually impossible to believe that Bena Bena males of any age suffer from confusion over their gender identity. This is not to say, however, that they enjoy being forcibly taken from their mothers for beatings, bloodlettings, and other physical abuses, or that they do not look upon childhood as a more favorable time in their lives. Indeed, why should they?

If the Oedipal hypothesis does not adequately explain the initiation rites we must look for other possibilities.[15] This is

[15]It must be pointed out that there are other objections to the views of Whiting and others. A study by Parker, Smith, and Ginat on a polygynous community in the United States did not support them (1975). Norbeck (1962), Young (1962), Cohen (1964), Honigmann (1967), and Kennedy (1970) have also questioned them.

not an easy task, as there are many questions that need to be asked of the existing ethnographic materials and their interpretations.

4

Some Comments on Exegeses

Themes that require consideration with respect to various accounts and interpretations of local exegeses include male rites of bloodletting, ideas about male and female maturation, genital mutilations, semen, secrecy, and the notion of symbolic birth or rebirth. Some Melanesian groups have extremely detailed beliefs about their ritual life (Poole 1981) while others, like the Bena Bena, apparently have very little by way of formal exegesis (Barth 1975).

I was never able to get a complete or entirely satisfactory explanation from Bena Bena informants as to just what they thought initiation ceremonies were all about. I did, however, get enough information to know that Bena Bena rites were very similar to Gahuku-Gama ones and, indeed, quite similar to those of other Eastern Highlanders as well. I was often told that the individuals who could truly explain these customs were no longer alive. I believe that was most probably the case, at least for Korofeigu. However, there are a number of questions that arise from the Bena Bena case which must be raised about the interpretations of local exegeses not only for the Bena Bena but for other New Guineans as well.

It has often been claimed, for example, that male bloodletting rites are a form of male menstruation. Unlike these cases (Allen 1967; Berndt 1962; Hogbin 1970; Lindenbaum 1976; Meigs 1976), and including the Gahuku-Gama (Read 1952), the Bena Bena deny that male bloodletting is the same as or even like menstruation (except insofar as they both involve bleeding). The Gnau of the West Sepik area likewise deny that their penis bleeding is like menstruation (Lewis 1980:2). The Ndumba also deny any connection between nosebleeding and menstruation. In their case (Hays and Hays 1982:221) and most others as we shall see, it was said to be done for the purpose of making the boys strong by cleansing them of "mothers' blood." This was also true among the Kuman (Nilles 1950:37). Interestingly, in some areas such as Awa (Newman and Boyd 1982), Ndumba (Hays and Hays 1982), and Auyana (Robbins 1982), girls also have their noses bled. This occurred among the Bena Bena as well. Berndt reports that for Kamano, Usurufa, Jale, and Fore puberty rites for girls include both nosebleeding and vaginal bleeding caused by the insertion of a wad of rough leaves (Berndt 1965:106). Among the Awa, bloodletting is apparently done to eliminate fluids in general and not specifically mother's blood (Newman and Boyd 1982:257). Although the Hua "make only a vague and partial identification between blood letting in general and menstruation," one of their healing rites is said to be a specific imitation of menstruation (Meigs 1976:398). The Bena Bena do make a connection between menstruation and the moon as do virtually all Highlanders and quite likely most Papua New Guineans in general.

But what does it mean to say that male bloodletting is menstruation? Does that mean it is *identical* to menstruation? An *imitation* of menstruation? *Similar* to menstruation? *Analogous* to menstruation? Is it simply a metaphor which they understand and we do not?[1] Furthermore, what does menstruation

[1] See Keesing on "Conventional Metaphors and Anthropological Metaphysics: The Problematic of Cultural Translation" (1985) for the difficulty in interpreting metaphors cross-culturally.

itself signify to the New Guineans compared to what it means for Europeans? As the claim that men imitate menstruation is a basis for the argument for the existence of womb envy (Bettelheim 1954; Lidz and Lidz 1989) it is worthy of some attention. Unfortunately, this is not an easy question to answer.

As far as I know the first mention of male bloodletting as menstruation in the New Guinea case appears in Kenneth Read's now classic article "The Nama Cult of the New Guinea Highlands." He says: "[Male] Initiation rites, in consequence, serve the same purpose for the male as menstruation for women. The one has been explained to me in terms of the other, and the same idea—the cyclical expulsion of blood—undoubtedly lies behind the men's ritual of nose bleeding" (1952:15). Ronald Berndt in *Excess and Restraint* says in one place that ". . . men themselves imitate the menstrual flow during certain ceremonies" (1962:57) and in another that "The periodic shedding of blood is also directly equated with female menstruation" (1962:98). Ian Hogbin, in *The Island of Menstruating Men,* says ". . . females regain their purity by natural menstruation, and men regain theirs by artificial menstruation" (1970:88). Philip Newman, writing of the Gururumba, says of the nosebleeding, "The resultant bloody flow is said to be equivalent to menstruation, and informants explicitly refer to the act as 'our (male) menstruation'" (1965:79). Then, over time, these statements are converted into ". . . male rituals of imitative menstruation" (Lindenbaum 1976:57).

It is not always clear whether these descriptions are the result of the purely emic statements of informants or if they are etic or some combination of both. This is an obvious and recurring problem in anthropological fieldwork and interpretation.[2]

[2] For a thoughtful and detailed discussion of the problems involved in interpreting ritual behavior in general and male menstruation in particular see Gilbert Lewis's *Day of Shining Red* (1980).

Similarly, what are we to make of the language involved? For Read the bloodletting "serves the same purpose." For Berndt it is both "imitative" and "equated with." In Hogbin's case it is "artificial," for Newman it is "equivalent," and for Lindenbaum it is "imitative" (in another place it is "mimicry" 1979:130), as it presumably must be, of course, for Bettelheim, Lidz and Lidz, and others, like Hiatt (1971), who subscribe to the notion of womb envy. There are multiple and very serious problems here: we do not know precisely what was asked of informants, what was actually told to the ethnographer, whether the translation is literal or interpretive, and we also do not know precisely what is meant by the descriptions offered in the English language. In Read's account quoted above, for example, he says "The one [male initiation rites] has been explained to me in terms of the other [menstruation for women]," but there is no account of precisely what he was told. Similarly, he says "the cyclical expulsion of blood—undoubtedly lies behind the men's ritual of nose bleeding" (1952:15). It seems clear that in this case the claim is simply Read's assumption.

Later in *The High Valley* he speaks of "the implicit envy of biological womanhood" (1965:155) which, again, raises the question of interpretation versus actual data. Consider also Tuzin's interpretation of bloodletting among Ilahita Arapesh:

> While cutting the penis is *probably* imitative of menstruation, and therefore a statement of the *enviability* of that function, the vaunting pride taken by the men in doing this to themselves proclaims the *transcendent power of masculinity*. In other words, women merely bleed; they are helpless creatures of their own sexuality, unable to govern or restrain their sexual energies (1980:77).[3]

One might well ask if women are truly helpless creatures, why would they be envied? In any case, as a result of these various claims and interpretations, we do not know from the available information if this might be truly considered womb

3 The emphases here, except for the word transcendent, are mine.

envy or not. A good case can be made on related grounds, however, that it is not.

The one thing that appears clear from virtually all of the ethnographic accounts is that the purpose of the bloodletting rites is specifically to rid oneself of female blood that is said to be polluting. "Among all female substances, menstrual blood is the most antithetical to all male substances and is highly polluting to both men *and* women" (Poole 1982:113). "But this [male] superiority is under constant threat from another substance, which this time flows exclusively and regularly from the woman's body, once Moon has pierced her and she has had her first period, namely, menstrual blood" (Godelier 1986:58). For the Tairora, "Menstrual blood is a major pollutant, potentially lethal to men not properly protected from its influence" (Watson 1983:320). Although Salisbury does not speak of pollution it is the mother's contribution (of blood) which must be diminished during the initiation rites (1962:34). Fore males fear menstrual pollution and cleanse themselves through initiation (Lindenbaum 1976, 1979) as, it appears, do most or all New Guineans who have such initiation rites.

It would seem that these male rites of bloodletting, claimed in some places to be menstruation, even if they are truly imitative of menstruation, not only cannot be interpreted as indicative of womb envy but are in fact the very opposite of that. Their purpose is to totally *rid* males of female blood. Indeed, from their point of view the purpose of menstruation even for females is to cleanse them of this highly dangerous and polluting substance. This is the very antithesis of womb envy. It can be seen most clearly perhaps in the Gururumba case:

> Similarly, life is produced by combining substances that contain it. These two substances are semen and womb-blood in the form of amorphous life principle, and semen in the form of vital material substance. Conception occurs when womb-blood is made solid and held in the body by semen, but menstruation occurs when it is not "solidified." In fact, menstrual blood

> becomes the antitheses of vital essence because it is regarded as dead womb-blood. . . .
>
> In a very important sense, vital essence is identified with sexual energy. This can be seen by examining a list of bodily substances thought to contain it as opposed to those which do not. It is in semen and womb-blood, the two substances involved in conception, but is not in menstrual blood or in other genital secretions such as urine . . . (Newman 1965:76).

The notion of menstrual blood being "dead womb blood" is found among the Gimi also and "Gimi women liken menstruation to a pregnancy which culminates in death rather than in the emergence of a separate, living child" (Gillison 1980:149). The Gimi case is further confused in that ". . . menstrual blood is held to be a part of the husband (transformed semen)" (A. Strathern 1996:75). The Sambia, too, distinguish between circulatory blood and womb blood (Herdt 1982b:196) and the latter is specifically antithetical to men. The Usen Barok distinguish between "clean blood" and menstrual blood (Wagner 1983:78).[4]

There is no indication anywhere in the literature that it is "womb blood" that is being imitated in the bloodletting rites and the evidence is overwhelming that it is polluting (menstrual-womb) blood that is at issue. The object of the bloodletting is to be rid of all female substances and qualities, not acquire them. Indeed, among the Awa the bleeding is specifically explained as helping to develop the *male* organs: "Bleeding the penis is explained to the initiates as similar, in this respect, to bleeding the nose but as contributing specifically to the strengthening and development of male reproductive organs" (Newman and Boyd 1982:257). This argument gains even more force when juxtaposed with other New Guinea beliefs about women in general, the vagina, the pain of childbirth, and also about fatherhood, to which we will return.

---

[4] Melanesian beliefs about blood would easily make a dissertation. The situation is further complicated by the fact that for the Usen Barok blood is used as a euphemism for semen (Wagner 1983:80).

To attempt to derive womb envy from the New Guinea materials is little more than a psychoanalytic fantasy. Gillison's explanation of men's presumed envy of females is an excellent example. Through a convoluted interpretation that involves, among other things, the equation of penis with flute, symbolic castration, the initiate acting as his own mother, then "giving birth to his own penis," the rite somehow implies an equivalence between the penis and the creativity of menstrual blood such that once menstrual blood is symbolically taken away from women through male rites of bloodletting its "phallic power is restored" (1980:164). I agree completely with Tuzin's (under)statement on this: "Thus, although the men may quip that their periodic cleansings are the 'male menstruation,' it would be too simple to infer that this merely represents male envy of female sexual parts or functions" (1980:77).

There is a similar problem here with respect to the issue of male pregnancy. In the case of the Hua, in spite of the fact that Meigs reports males saying, "No, our pregnancy claim is just talk" (1976:393), and in spite of the fact that *kupa* (male pregnancy) is a "feared and abhorred condition" (p. 397), she claims that men claim to be pregnant because "they appear to possess a will to believe they are fertile" (p. 397). As everywhere in New Guinea, as far as I know, infertility is always blamed on females rather than males, this would appear to me a strange claim. This is all the more so because among the Hua, as elsewhere, ". . . Ostensibly, the sexes are alike in loathing the processs of menstruation and child birth as disgusting and dangerous" (p.393).

There is a problem with respect to the position of blood in New Guinea belief systems which can merely be mentioned here. This is, again, a question of interpretation. More often than not when blood is reported as a significant element in ritual procreation, no distinction is made between one form of blood and another. However, just as the Gururumba and Gimi distinguish womb blood from menstrual blood, so the Ok distinguish between at least two kinds of blood: "The shared substance between members of a clan is generally conceptualized as blood, but this is the living blood in one's arteries and is thought of as categorically distinct from menstrual blood, so no ambiguity arises. With respect to nourishing the foetus, on the other hand, it is also commonly claimed that repeated acts of intercourse are necessary to cause birth because the foetus also requires the nourishment of male semen until it has grown large enough so the quickening of life can be felt—after which intercourse should be discontinued" (Barth 1987:13). Meigs, on the other hand, claims that the Hua do not distinguish between the blood let in bloodlettings and menstrual blood in spite of the fact that "Blood let from the limbs of middle-aged men was eaten by other males to enhance growth and strength" (1984:57)! The Gnau, who both eat blood and smear it on children, have rather complicated beliefs about blood which, among other things, appear to distinguish between mother's brother's blood and the blood you are born with, between father's blood and his younger brother's blood, and so on (Lewis 1975:37). It is interesting to note here that when blood passes from mother's brother to sister's son it is regarded as a transmission of positive *male* life force (A. Strathern 1996:68, my emphasis). Similarly, the mother's blood among the Daribi is "that of her own brother" which, again, seems to me to represent the transmission of male substance (A. Strathern 1996:71).

The Sambia, as above, make a distinction between different types of blood as well: ". . . there is a tacit distinction that amounts to the difference between circulatory blood and menstrual-womb blood. Both males and females possess circulatory blood (*menjaaku*); but only females have menstrual blood (*chenchi*), categorized with all female contamination" (Herdt 1982b:196).[5] According to Ivan Mbaginta'o, a young man from

5 In the Sambia case, if only females have menstrual blood, it would obviously be difficult to interpret male bloodletting as imitative of menstruation.

Herdt's general research area who actually experienced the initations, ". . . The blood from the nose was allowed to fall into the stream, to flow to the Papuan plains. When the blood of the uninitiated boys had flowed out of sight, we, theoretically, received new blood. The blood from the nose represented our mothers' birth blood" (1971:290). The Karavarans, too, make a distinction between different kinds of blood: "There is an unarticulated distinction between the unconfined and polluting sexual blood of women and the normally confined, nonpolluting nonsexual blood common to both men and women" (Errington 1974:611). Among the Fore and others, "The blood is a libation to the Creative Beings and to the ancestral spirits of the lineage. It is an offering to insure their spiritual patronage so that they will sustain the 'giver.'" (Berndt 1962:98). Bimin-Kuskusmin, too, distinguish between different types of blood—male blood as contrasted with female blood, for example, but also apparently between male blood transmitted through females and menstrual blood (Poole 1984:197). The Bush Mekeo apparently distinguish between bilateral blood relationship and agnatic blood relationship as well as between male and female blood (Mosco 1983:27).[6] According to Mead, the Mountain Arapesh distinguish between "good blood and bad blood" (1940:349). Among the Orokaiva they distinguish "male blood," which is transmitted by a man to his son, from the blood women receive (Schwimmer 1969:132).[7] The Gnau make a distinction

6 It is not entirely clear just what Mosco has in mind when speaking of "bloods." Consider this passage from his work: ". . . With sexual reproduction, father and mother begin or conceive a child with the mixing of their sexual bloods—semen (*ilaila*) and womb blood (*ifa inainga*) respectively—in equal proportions in the 'abdomen' (*ina*) of the mother." Does this mean semen is regarded as a form of blood? Similarly, as he speaks of "womb blood" does this imply another kind of blood? Given the confusion here what does it mean to say that "In any case, each child receives half its hereditary blood from its father, half from its mother?" This is especially problematic when he also claims that ". . . the father's semen 'dries,' 'solidifies' or 'coagulates' (*engonfo*) the mother's 'wet' and 'fluid' or 'amorphous' *(ekome)* womb blood to form the child." Thus, even if the child does get half from each parent the contributions are not similar.

7 Given the potential complexity of Papua New Guineans' beliefs about blood one would have

between stagnant blood and blood that moves (Lewis 1980:152). The Foi distinguish between "blood held in the uterus by an accumulation of semen," and "menstrual blood which a woman releases during her period, blood which has not been 'fastened' by an accumulation of semen . . ." (Glass 1995:166).

Questions having to do with blood are much more complex than they appear to be in the literature. Feil, for example, says: "Among Chimbu, Kuma and Narak, idioms of blood unite people in many complex ways but it is never purged, ignored or overridden by male influence or interference . . . .

"Blood is most often viewed in these societies and those further west as originating with the mother, as flowing from her and her group . . . the incontrovertable fact is that, in Wahgi societies and those further west, we encounter for the first time female idioms of blood applied to important, lasting relations" (1987:159–160). It is by no means clear why these are "female idioms" any more than male. O'Hanlon and Frankland make what I believe is an important point here:

> The second idiom, that of blood (*na maiam*) is one of some complexity but one of the primary referents of "my blood" (*na maiam*) is ego's MB. The employment of blood as an idiom to denote ego's link to his mother and her agnates is, of course, a commonplace of Highlands ethnography. A primary manifestation of this is the assertion in the conception dogma of a number of Highlands peoples that it is specifically the mother who contributes blood to the formation of the foetus . . . . The Wahgi case is more complex. While the phrase describing conception, *maiam se dale,* does literally mean "blood placing becoming", the Wahgi do not say whose blood this is. When pressed they tend to state generally that the blood is both that of the mother and the father . . . . This in turn seems consistent with the fact that *maiam* as an idiom to denote MB may *also* be extended to cover parental maternal kin—the subgroups of MM, FM, MMM, and FFM. . . . In this extended usage ego is being

to question Feil's perhaps oversimplified claim for the Wahgi and others: ". . . Whatever the explanation, the incontrovertible fact is that, in Wahgi societies and those further west, we encounter for the first time female idioms of blood applied to important, lasting relations. Blood is culturally emphasized, not debased, and individuals are subject to and finally aligned with other than narrow, unilateral and tightly bounded entities "(1987:160).

> related to two of these groups by blood traced through the male line. The men of all these groups are additionally felt to possess the same influence that is exercised over ego by his MB (or possibly a more diffuse version of it) (1986:186).

Blood can even be ritually transformed as in this case from the Ilahita Arapesh: ". . . Unknown to the boys, as they are feeling around in the mud and silt for the nonexistent shell, they are contaminating themselves with the 'oily essence' of their own penile blood, which supposedly has adhered to the bottom of the stream . . . . In the days that the blood essences have lain on the stream-bed they have mingled with the spiritual presences already there—the invisible potencies of ancestral shades, cult spirits, and *maolinipunemb* figures. In short, the blood which carried away pernicious feminine influences now comes back to the novices charged with superlatively *masculine* influences. The youths have met and interacted with the world of spirits by the medium of their own body essences, certifying in the act their office as complete males" (Tuzin 1980:72–73). Whitehead says of this: "Here blood, suitably transformed through ritual operations, is acting as the equivalent of semen in the south" (1986:88). Transformed blood is also reported elsewhere in New Guinea (Lewis 1980:174–75; Mead 1940–41:348–349; Gillison 1980:164).

Among the Bumbita Arapesh menstruation and penis bleeding are considered "equivalents." However, Leavitt goes on to explain:

> . . . [A] woman rids herself of "bad blood" through her period, and a man does the same thing by cutting his penis. However, because men and women are different types of beings, the purification processes are quite different. First, the bad blood held responsible for fatigue, malaise and weakness has different origins in men and women. For women, bad blood builds up naturally as a byproduct of their feminine maturation—a woman's bad blood is her "poison". . . By contrast, bad blood develops in men mostly as a result of their own actions, through associating with bad blood's two sources: food and women . . . Second, purification is different in men and women because of the initiative involved with penis bleeding.

One of Leavitt's informants

> . . . describes menstruation as a woman's "sickness" while penis bleeding is a man's "breath," by which he means that it is his source of new vigor and vitality (Leavitt 1991:900).

One might well wonder how these different practices can truly be seen as equivalent, except for the fact that they both involve bloodletting.

The relative importance of blood vis-à-vis semen is not always clear. Thus, for example, Newman reports that among the Gururumba semen is a relatively passive substance which is "eaten" by the womb blood (1989), not the impression one has of semen elsewhere in the literature.[8] However, the Gururumba also keep small pieces of quartz which are rubbed on the initiates and then put in the open end of the sacred flutes. They say this is "feeding the flutes" and the quartz is "like semen." Pig fat is also equated with the crystals and hence with semen as well (Newman 1989).

Another widespread belief held by the Bena Bena as well as other New Guineans, is that boys do not mature as quickly or as easily as girls and require special ritual attention to properly do so (Herdt 1982; Read 1952). Like the Gahuku-Gama, they emphasized during male initiations that the youths should grow up quickly or their wives would not "wait for them." In order to bring this about they separated the initiates from females at different periods of time, imposed certain food taboos, at times gave them special foods, performed rites of bloodletting and cane swallowing, and subjected them to harsh beatings, sleep deprivation, overheating, cold, and so on. They also emphasized repeatedly the dangers of associating too much with women, the polluting qualities of menstrual blood, the particular dangers of sexual intercourse, the importance of regularly performing the cleansing rites, and the superiority of males in general. The belief that boys do

---

8 There may be a question of interpretation involved here as to say in Melanesian pidgin that something eats something (*em i kai kai em*) does not necessarily render that something as passive. *Kai kai* also means merely to incorporate something. To eat can also be a euphemism for intercourse.

not mature naturally as do girls is widespread in New Guinea and has been reported as local exegesis by Buchbinder and Rappaport (1976), Herdt (1981), Poole (1982), Read (1952), and many others.

While it is apparently true that girls before adolescence do have a growth spurt and seem to overtake boys (Malcolm 1966, 1970, 1970a; Sinnet 1971; Sinnet and Whyte 1973), just why this should have become so salient for Highlands cultures is somewhat questionable. First, boys do, for example, start with an advantage in height and weight and they also achieve higher stature at a later age (Malcolm 1970:35). New Guinea belief systems for some reason ignore this and fix on the pre-adolescent pattern. As above, it is interesting to consider Read's original statement on this point: "They [Gahuku-Gama] recognize, indeed, that in physiological endowment men are inferior to women, and, characteristically, they have recourse to elaborate artificial means to redress the contradiction and to demonstrate its opposite. A girl's growing breasts and her first menstruation are signs of a maturing process which is without obvious parallel in the boy, a fact that the men resent. Betrothals are often broken off because the girl has outstripped the boy in physical growth . . ." (1952:15).

Here again, it is not very clear what is meant precisely by physiological inferiority. Presumably it is because the girls seem to grow faster than boys during their preadolescence. This is connected to the fact that girls menstruate and boys do not. But as menstruation occurs very late in New Guinea females, between 17 to 19 years of age (Buchbinder 1973:75; Malcolm 1970: 51; Gray 1982), it is not clear how this would explain the preadolescent growth spurt. Similarly, Read asserts there are no "obvious parallels" in male development with respect to the development of secondary sex characteristics. But this is simply not so. Boys do experience scrotal and testicular enlargement, develop facial and body hair, penile enlargement, and their voices begin to change (Malcolm 1970:32). Furthermore, in his study of the Bundi, Malcolm found that the attainment of adolescence occurs for boys at 18.9 years whereas the onset of menarche in girls is at 18.8, hardly an indication of greater delay in boys, although obviously both Bundi girls and boys are considerably delayed by international standards (1966:18). As this delay appears to be related to nutrition and is as well perhaps genetic, and as most of the Highlanders have not been studied, it is possible that these figures would not hold for all. In any case, even if it were true that boys matured somewhat slower than girls, the Highlanders could have simply changed the relative ages of betrothed couples so that wives were somewhat younger than husbands. Indeed, in many cases they were. Hays has suggested that it may be the timing here that is important. That is, the girls' growth spurt comes earlier and the boys' later which may well reinforce their beliefs about the differences in maturation (Hays 1994). There is another perhaps related factor here that needs to be considered, the ubiquitous practices having to do with the penis.

Male genital mutilation has been of interest to anthropologists for quite some time. Even now, however, there is little understanding of this widespread practice. LeTourneau regarded circumcision as a substitute for human sacrifice (1893). Zaborowski pointed out in 1896 that circumcision at puberty marked the entrance to adult social life. He also believed that circumcision and castration were two different phenomena. Frazer thought that circumcision separated an individual from a vital portion of himself that would later be treated supernaturally (1904). Briffault (1927) suggested that circumcision was an attempt to imitate female genital defloration. Westermarck (1926) claimed it was a means for making a boy into a man capable of procreation and marriage. Crawley (1927) regarded it as a means of preventing the retention of magically dangerous secretions and also as the sacrificing of a part in order to guarantee the well-being of the whole. Bryk (1934) attempted to explain circumcision as a substitute for castration and human sacrifice. It has also been explained as having to do with either increased or decreased sensuality, as a prevention of pederasty and onanism, for increased fertility, endurance, and cleanliness. Numerous medical and hygenic reasons have also been offered (Bryk 1934). Freud, of course, Zaborowski notwithstanding, maintained that circumcision was a form of castration (1939). Bettelheim viewed genital mutilations as attempts to emulate the female genitals (1954). Van Gennep considered circumcision to be of social rather than physiological importance (1960). For Burton and Whiting genital mutilations are viewed as separating the child from the mother and helping to resolve identity conflict (1961). Young regarded genital mutilations as a dramatization of the male sex role thus differentiating the sexes (1962).

Harrington argued that there are three types of genital mutilation—circumcision, supercision, and subincision—which had not been clearly separated. When these were separated he found at that "Circumcision is associated with high sexual differentiation in socialization practices, and societies that supercise are likely to have low sexual differentiation, even controlling for region of the world" (1968:955). Graber has more recently argued, following Reik (1975), that ". . . fathers project hostility toward their own fathers onto their sons," which then leads to genital mutilation. He also argued that "cultures having both patrilocality and the state should be especially likely to practice male genital mutilation . . ." (1981:428).

About the only thing these different positions have in common is their lack of extensive data and consequent divorce from reality. Indeed, in his review of circumcision customs Bryk was led to conclude that the explanations given, ". . . furnish a splendid example of the versatility of human extravagant imagination, and are, at the same time, a document of the ambivalent validity of casuistic argumentation" (quoted in Crapanzano 1982:19). Harrington was quite right when he said circumcision, supercision, and subincision had not been clearly separated. But even his tripartite scheme does not accomodate all varieties of genital practices. For example, the Bena Bena and others shot a miniature stone-pointed arrow repeatedly into the urethra to draw blood. Garia did essentially the same thing but with a thorn-headed arrow ". . . so padded that it cannot penetrate deeply" (Lawrence 1984:208). The Wogeo cut the glans with a sharp crab claw (Hogbin 1970). The Awa cut wedges out of each side of the glans with a bamboo knife (Newman and Boyd 1982) as, apparently, did the Kwoma (Whiting and Reed 1938:196).

Ilahita Arapesh rub penes and scrota with stinging nettles and lacerate the penis with bamboo knives (Tuzin 1982:338). They also repeatedly insert barbed grass stems into the urethra (Tuzin 1980:74). Abelam fathers tell their sons to strike their penes with nettles to rid them of "bad blood" and later, during initiations, their penes are "incised" (Kaberry 1941a:361). This was apparently done with a sharp piece of quartz (Hauser-Schaublin 1995:40). Among the Eastern Highlanders Berndt reported on a length of "spear" grass treated with ashes is shoved into the penis, withdrawn, and then a twig inserted which is twirled around until the youth cries in pain and urinates (1962:98). Manam boys were taught to insert long thin reeds or other sharp objects into their penes to draw blood (Bohm 1983:81). The Kwoma scrape the initiates' penes with stinging nettles (Whiting 1941:67). The Murik taught the "secret skill of urethral insertion drew blood from the initiates' penes and rubbed their bodies with it" (Barlow and Lipset 1990:17). The Gnau traditionally forced a sharp wallaby bone "into the dorsum of the penis just above the glans" and, after contact, began to use razor blades to bleed their penes (Lewis 1980:78). Circumcision and subincision apparently do not occur in most of Melanesia.[9]

[9] It is not very clear in some cases precisely what is done to the male genitals. For example, Powdermaker uses the term "circumcision" to describe what is done to youths on Lesu but, while it is clear that some kind of cutting was done, she did not actually observe the procedure nor, apparently, did she ask about it in detail (1971). Burridge, too, speaks of circumcision among the Tangu (1969:172) but gives no description of what actually occurs. I believe it is

Surely such a widespread and seemingly absurd act as abusing the penis in these bizarre ways requires a very basic kind of explanation. I suggest there may be one having to do with the normal male anatomy. In spite of over a century of interest on this subject, so far as I know no one has apparently considered there might be a more practical explanation for "abusing" the male genitals, nor has anyone considered the condition of the normal uncircumcised penis.[10] At birth the prepuce is actually attached to the glans and is still developing. This means that the normal prepuce of the newborn is still nonretractable. During the first few years of life and lasting in some cases until as late as age 17, the foreskin slowly becomes fully retractable. While this is a natural process it can be hurried through early masturbation or sex although this can be painful. In some cases the foreskin does not fully retract even by age 17 (Gairdner 1949; Oster 1968). In such cases one operation that can be performed involves simply making a slit in the foreskin. It is not completely unusual for teenaged boys to actually be circumcised because of this type of problem.

Even if a boy develops normally he can still have a tight foreskin which, although retractable with a bit of effort, can be relatively difficult and painful. Furthermore, the glans is extremely sensitive as the function of the foreskin is to protect it. Forcing the foreskin to retract can bring about scarring and create problems. Thus first attempts at intercourse can end in failure and even when successful can involve considerable pain.[11]

---

highly unlikely that circumcision as such was actually performed. Gray, too, mentions "male circumcision" but I believe she is referring to the treatment of the penis in general (1991:78).

[10]I find this incredible although it is apparently true. Furthermore, as far as I have been able to find out, no one has ever interviewed a random sample of uncircumcised males with respect to their initial and early sexual behavior.

[11]Glasse reports a Huli custom that may be relevant to this point: "Before copulating for the first time, the husband pours foul smelling tree oil on his wife's vulva, for the genitals of a virgin are 'hot' and may damage his penis" (1968:59). It could also be the case that the tightness of the virginal vagina and hymen makes first intercourse more difficult for both males and females.

Consider this account from one of Leavitt's interviewees:

> . . . He points out that his ignorance of the sexual act was indicative of a larger concern over coping with the marriage. He then continued by saying that for some time the sexual act was actually painful. He put in [sic] these terms: "When my cock was hard and I had sex with her, this bone of hers, the meat of the woman's genitals, it pressed on my cock. It rubbed on it and made it heavy. I wanted to have sex with the woman, but it was too heavy, too painful." This description would be of little consequence if it were not for the fact that his language here mirrors an earlier description he made of a ritual procedure performed by adolescents to prepare their bodies for the onset of sexual relations. When Bumbita males reach their early teens, they make a small incision into a part of the foreskin (*prepuce frenulum*) at the glans on the underside of their penes. This procedure is performed only once and is considered entirely different from the usual hygienic bloodletting. People claim that this procedure is necessary for the successful performance of the sex act (1991:902).

Given this situation, could it not be related to the problem of delayed maturation as perceived by the New Guinea Highlanders? If boys are reticent about having sex, whether because of their physical condition or cultural beliefs, or both, it becomes understandable why girls might not wish to wait for them or, indeed, might make fun of them. It would hardly do for dominant and forceful males to be unable to adequately perform the sex act. And, if older males are aware of these problems, is it not conceivable that they might attempt to ritually address them? Consider, for example, that superincision (also called supercision) as practiced by some Melanesians involves cutting a slit in the foreskin (Chowning 1987:134; Layard 1942). This is also a common procedure for the Tikopians, in Tonga (Firth 1963:383-88), in Tahiti (Levy 1973:117), in parts of Indonesia (Hollan 1990), and quite likely in other areas as well. The Tahitians claim to do this primarily for cleanliness but, interestingly enough, they also say that "sexual activity might split an uncut foreskin" (Levy 1973:119). Among the Abelam, the penis of a newly wed man is cut "during his first intense period of sexual intercourse with his wife" ostensibly "to release polluted blood. . . ." (Hauser-Schaublin

1995:40). The Awa conceive of penis bleeding as "contributing specifically to the strengthening and development of male reproductive organs" (Newman and Boyd 1982:257). The penis blood from Ilahita Arapesh initiates is collected in leaves which are then tucked under the bark of large trees so that "As the tree grows strong and great, so will the novice" (Tuzin 1982:338). Berndt reported that "The insertion of objects into the penis duct is said to make the penis itself strong; for if this is strong, so will be the arrows he shoots . . ." (1962:100).[12] He also reports that "The man with a strong penis is a strong warrior" (1962:108). Although it is not entirely clear it appears that "circum-incision" among the Big Nambas of the New Hebrides is to make the male organ grow strong (Layard 1942:486). The Garia performed penile incision "to guarantee that they become sexually attractive men" (Lawrence 1984:208). Supercision is directly linked to sexual maturity among the Toraja of Indonesia: "Like scarification of the forearm in more recent times, supercision is consciously viewed as a means of marking male adulthood, but in addition to representing physical courage, strength, and boldness, supercision also explicitly marks sexual maturity and virility (or its potential)" (Hollan and Wellenkamp 1990: 22). And, "By undergoing supercision, one demonstrates the minimal amount of courage and boldness necessary to validate one's male identity. One is also thought to be (or have the potential to become) sexually potent and virile enough to satisfy the sexual needs of women and to father children" (Hollan and Wellenkamp 1990:23). It is at least suggestive that among Sambia the "birth" of the glans penis occurs at puberty (Herdt 1990:28). Could it be the case that when older Sambia initiates "get the go-ahead to 'relax their tight penises'" (Herdt

[12] That the foreskin plays some role in the attention given to the male genitals during initiation rites might also be seen in the fact that when Berndt's initiates approached the place of initiation they see an adult male (the "guardian of the flutes") with his foreskin pierced by an arrow and thereby pinned to a piece of sugar cane (1962:171). Also see Juillerat (1992:56) for a brief discussion of ritual treatment of the foreskin.

1982a:57), the elders are speaking literally? Similarly suggestive, perhaps, is that penis mutilations are completely absent from those cultures in which fellatio is cited as a form of ritual homosexuality.[13] Oral sex might be seen in this context as having the same function as the various other practices with respect to the penis (the preparation of the penis for intercourse?). Could this be one of those male secrets that would shame men if women knew?[14]

Related to this is the Sambia belief that males do not naturally produce semen (Herdt 1981:204) and the beliefs of other New Guineans that men have only a finite supply which can be depleted (Newman, 1965:77).[15] While we know these beliefs are not true, we recognize that cultural beliefs are not always rational or irrational and may be simply nonrational (Shweder 1984:28). But it would be all too easy to just let it go at that. Whether irrational or nonrational these beliefs are part of a reasonably consistent theory of human life and development. This semen-depletion theory holds that semen is the crucial element in the formation and continuance of life, that it can be lost or depleted, particularly through too much sexual activity, that this can result in sickness and death, and that men must perform various rituals to insure this does not happen. If men believe this, then their behavior with respect to females "makes sense," as does the homosexuality that occurs among Sambia and some others. All this makes sense however irra-

[13] Herdt maintains that ". . . penis cutting is absent from (RH) [ritualized homosexuality] groups" but acknowledges at the same time that circum-incision is present in the New Hebrides where they practice anal intercourse (1984b:67).

[14] The people around Mount Hagen do not mutilate or abuse the penis, but they apparently employ magic to make the penis strong: "Meanwhile, four old men cooked a single small pig in the *tumb* enclosure. They told me: 'Young men should not come here. If they do, their penises will be soft and weak and they will not be able to copulate with their wives and beget children. They should stay by the *porembil*, which is long like an erect penis, and cook pigs there.' The phallic import of the *porembil* stake was thus clearly pointed out; and on receiving this explanation I retired from the *tumb* enclosure" (Strathern 1970:582).

[15] The Sambia beliefs about males being unable to produce semen are somewhat difficult to understand given that, of course, they do, but also because of the production of smegma which occurs even in young boys and is often mistaken for semen.

tional or nonrational the initial premises may be, and however lost in antiquity the origins, and thus the beliefs are not only perpetuated but apparently form the very basis for Highlands religious systems. I will return to this later.

The homosexuality that has been reported for some New Guinea groups (Godelier 1986; Herdt 1981, 1984; Kelly 1977; Landtman 1927; Schieffelin 1982; Van Baal 1966; Williams 1936) is in a sense only one relatively trivial element within the much larger context of New Guinea initiation rites and their attendant belief systems. This is particularly true in the case of the Highlands because ritualized homosexuality is overwhelmingly a lowlands Papua New Guinea phenomena except in rather peripheral Northern Anga groups like the Sambia and Baruya (Herdt 1984), and does not otherwise occur in the New Guinea Highlands. But even when considering the whole of New Guinea, homosexuality, whether it be oral or anal, is merely one means of several to a much larger end, namely, the transmission of semen from generation to generation and in perpetuity.

Whereas homosexuality exists only in some groups, the beliefs about semen and various means of employing it in ritual exist everywhere. Thus the Bimin-Kuskusmin engage in collective masturbation and place tubes of semen among phallocrypt gourds and in taro gardens for the patrilineal transmission of the vital substance (Poole 1982:106). Similarly:

> . . . fleshy parts of the body are associated with the female contribution, with certain exceptions that are associated with the male contribution. All passages involved in breathing, hearing, and seeing (all associated with bony structure and key ritual "sense"); the accumulation of "sacred male knowledge" (transmitted through the frontal cranial sutures); and the flow of both semen and fertile fluids (but not menstrual blood), are believed to emanate from the paternal procreative contribution. Thus, the female anatomy (and the female foods that sustain it) is considered temporary, illness-prone, and weak. It is associated with the more contaminating of human wastes and is largely antithetical to ritual efficacy (Poole 1981:127).

At first menses the Gimi "'force' her [the bride] to drink

'ancestral semen' (water taken from a river owned by her husband's clan) and to eat a 'spirit child' (a possum shot in the husband's clan forest and encased in sugarcane and vines, symbolic of the penis)" (Gillison 1980:159). The Bena Bena use a mixture of semen, soot, and blood to paint part of the adult male costume which they give to their sons at initiation (Langness 1974). Among the Foi the semen of older men was rubbed into the navels of the immature initiates (J. Weiner 1988:22). The Kimam rub semem into incisions made in the initiate's arms, legs, and abdomen (Serpenti 1965:164). In other groups such as the Marind-anim the youths are fed dishes "garnished with sperm" (quoted in Herdt 1984:25). The Marind-anim rubbed semen on their unmarried girls as well (Van Baal 1966:155), and human sperm was "widely applied in fertility magic" (1966:194). "Among the Gebusi, a male child is fed his father's semen at the age of eighteen to twenty-four months in order to ensure his early growth" (Kelly 1993:149). While homosexuality is an important topic in its own right, it clearly should not as such be the primary focus for the understanding of male initiations. As far as I can determine there are few, if any, New Guinea cultures that do not believe in some form of the semen-depletion theory and/or the importance of semen in general.[16]

The Northern Tairora, for example, believe of semen that "As a key stuff in the creation of a human being, semen contributes, obviously, to [their] views regarding males as the primary if not unique progenitors of their offspring, while the female procreative role is stereotyped as secondary, even am-

[16]Hays has suggested that perhaps the beliefs about semen depletion arise from the fact that most males cannot have sex repeatedly without waiting for some period of time between ejaculations. In any case, beliefs about semen depletion seem to be widespread even outside of Papua New Guinea. Balzac, for example, believed in such a theory: "... he [Balzac] firmly believed that every man had at birth a finite store of vital fluid and that the secret of creative life was to hoard one's energy. Sperm was for him an emission of pure cerebral substance—once, after having spent the night with an enchanting creature, he turned up at the house of a friend, crying: 'I just lost a book!'" These views were apparently common in China as well (Leys:23).

bivalent, above all in connection with male offspring" (Watson 1983:258). For the Kimam

> . . . sperm is believed to contain great powers. It is an excellent medicine against illness. Just as by cohabitation a man may with his sperm produce life and cause his vitality to pass into that of his child, so it is thought possible to cause the outstanding characteristics of great cultivators and head-hunters to pass into the children in the *burawa* (Serpenti 1965:164).

The Gururumba identify semen as "vital essence" (Newman 1965:76). The Foi believe that "Whereas women produce menstrual blood spontaneously and regularly, the stock of semen in a man's body is depleted during sexual intercourse. In order to replenish it, men must eat the fat and juices of meat, for it is only meat that the body transforms into semen" (J. Weiner 1988:41). The Daribi have similar beliefs about eating meat. In addition they observe: "When a man wants to have intercourse, the flow of *kawa* [semen] from all over his body causes an erection in his penis; after it has been ejaculated, according to Daribi, the skin becomes slack. It is for this reason that the flesh of young men is sleek and firm, whereas that of old men hangs loosely on their bones" (Wagner 1972:41). Schieffelin says of the Kaluli:

> While the female is enervating and debilitating, the male embodies the qualities of productivity, vigor, stimulation, and energy. This male influence is concentrated in semen. Semen has a kind of magical quality that promotes physical growth and mental understanding. A youngster going to stay in a foreign area may be fed a mixture of semen, salt, and ginger to stimulate him to learn the language quickly. By the same reasoning, frequent repeated sexual intercourse is felt to be necessary to invigorate a child in the womb. (When not looking to produce children Kaluli avoid sex, lest a man dissipate his energy.) Semen is also necessary for young boys to attain full growth to manhood (Schieffelin 1976:124).

In some areas adultery causes "semen out of place" that can bring about sickness in both the adulterous wife and her husband (A. Strathern 1996:18). Among the Bimin-Kuskusmin wild boar's fat is the symbol for semen: "Bimin-Kuskusmin . . . use wild boar's fat in their initiation rituals as the essential symbol for semen; they inaugurate phases of their rituals by burning/exploding containers of such fat/semen, and they anoint their novices, and their taro plants in the sacred gardens, with it. Thus a creature of great inherent interest to members of the congregation is linked as a concrete symbol to the vast theme of man-taro equivalence and the male's fertilizing role in gardening and human growth" (Barth 1987:36).

The most detailed list of the uses of semen can be found in Van Baal's *Dema*:

> A more interesting feature is the serving of the novices with food mixed with sperma. Sperma plays a dominant part in the Marind-anim pharmacopoeia. Wirz mentions the following applications: smearing it on wounds and sores makes them heal rapidly; swallowing it is good for the stomach; in the festive sago-dish sperma is often secretly mixed with the food to stimulate the men who are going to partake in promiscuous sexual intercourse during the ensuing dance; a young man who covets a certain girl will hand her some tidbit which he first mixed with his sperma. Applied to natural objects, sperma makes them last longer. When in the myth of *Wariop* and *Sapai* a new tree grows from *Sapai's* mutilated body, the men carve grooves into the bark of the tree and rub them with sperma to give the tree more stamina. Sperma fixes the black pigment on the teeth and lends permanence to the scarifications of the girls. It promotes the fertility of the crops and must be applied to the buds and the eyes. It is frequently applied to the *wati.* It is also put on the leaf sheaths of cocounut and sago palms. To that end fertility rites are organized which have much in common with the rites to dispel sickness. In both cases a [usually limited, V. B.] number of women have intercourse with as many men as possible, while the excreta are collected in a coconut-bowl. In the case of a fertility rite the sperma is applied to the plants; when the rite serves to dispel sickness, part of the fluid is smeared on the bodies of all the members of the group, and the remainder mixed with food (Van Baal 1966:547–8).

The Marind-anim may be extreme in their beliefs about the power of semen. Van Baal continues on this theme: ". . . Fertility is before all a matter of sperma. Sperma is the essence of life, of permanence, of health and prosperity. Living beings can be born from sperma even outside the womb.

A live wallaby is born from an emission of semen in *Aramemb's* girdle-shell; *Ugu* originates from the sperma spilled on *Harau's* mat during the *otiv-bombari* held in celebration of her marriage; yams grow out of *Aramemb's* head and shoulders after he has anointed his body with sperma; *Yano* makes living wallabies by smearing slices of wallaby-meat with sperma; bananas grow out of *Geb's* wounds after they have been treated with sperma. . . . Sperma is the essence of life and every ceremony leads to the effusion of sperma. . . . The role of the women in the procreative process is too conspicuous to be entirely ignored, but the Marind are fully convinced that it is the male sex whose function is definitely preponderant" (1966:817). Marie Reay, looking back upon her fieldwork, says of Kuma: "Nearly thirty years later, reading Herdt (1981), I wondered about the only part of the male initiation that I did not observe. This was an excursion into the forest, where the boys had to play the flutes and jump over logs. At the time I had been awake for two consecutive days and nights and, although invited to come along, I was too exhausted and went home to bed. But in 1981 I reflected that the augmentation of semen would be consistent with the Kuma males' ambition to make babies from that substance alone" (1992:156). Although he does not discuss it in detail it is clear from Lewis's account of the Gnau that semen is importantly involved in the creation of a fetus and somehow can be converted into blood (1980:174).

Sperm can feature only symbolically in some areas: "The chief product associated with miraculous physical growth among Orokaiva is the coconut, which is marked as a male fruit. Men will carry pairs of coconuts, tied together so as to resemble a phallus (the stalks represent the penis and the nuts the testicles). Oil from these coconuts, extracted by the women, is copiously applied to the novices' bodies. I have elsewhere shown that Orokaiva see this substance as a vegetable equivalent of sperm (Schwimmer 1974)" (Schwimmer 1984:260).

As elsewhere, the Bena Bena initiation ceremonies were described as a male secret. Women and uninitiated boys were said to be forbidden to view them under penalty of death. The Bena Bena, like the Gahuku-Gama, do not state that the rites or the sacred *nama* flutes originally belonged to women, although it is possible they may have had such a belief. I never heard anyone in Bena Bena suggest that women would laugh at them if they knew about the rites although Read reports this for Gahuku (1952:6).

Although I do not have detailed information about all of the above I am certain that they are similar in their important fundamentals to the practices of many other New Guinea groups. There are many unanswered questions that still need to be raised here. For example, what of the secrecy? Read in his now classic early paper asserted the whole ritual complex was basically a charade (1952:8), that women knew the secrets, or at least some of them, but went along with them anyway. And given the fact that older women, those past childbearing age, were not expected to look away when the flute processions passed, they must have known at least that the sounds did not emanate from gigantic birdlike monsters or the like. Similarly, it seems to me most unlikely that no one *ever* disclosed any of the secrets to women.[17] Among the Kwoma, ". . . The men tell the women and the uninitiated youths that the sounds of gongs, sacred flutes, bull-roarers, and the great water gong are made by daimons [sic]. Although the women and youths pretend to believe, they actually know that men are producing such sounds" (Whiting and Reed 1938:192). Furthermore, women *did* participate in the rites at least at some times. For example, the women's ritual attack on the initiation party. Berndt suggests that for Kamano, Usurufa, Jale, and Fore:

> . . . Men play the executive role in ritual, but it is a co-operative

[17]One Bena Bena woman with whom I worked confessed to me that some of the women did know the secrets but would not disclose them to her because they were afraid the men would be angry.

> undertaking. They keep various ritual objects secret, particularly the flutes, but their use in ritual necessarily brings in women. Women's use of the term co-wife for the flute indicates the closeness of their involvement and incidentally tells us something about their attitude toward men's ritual, for the co-wife relationship is notoriously one of strain. Women are acquainted not only with the cosmological knowledge and the secondary myths but also with nearly all the sacred mythology, including accounts of creation, even if they are not aware of all the symbolic meanings. Only certain sections of ritual and some of the objects, as well as esoteric explanations, remain the special possession of men. But even here women surreptitiously know much of what goes on (1965:95).

Among the Ndumba, women dress the youths for their initiation, prepare food for them, dance at various stages of the rites, and also participate in a mock attack (1982:211).

Whiting and Reed report that for the Kwoma, ". . . The dances which mark the investiture of youths are attended by the women and are occasions of ceremonial licence. During the dance women give small tokens to men of their choice signifying their desire for sexual intercourse. Women may not have intercourse with boys of the youngest age-grade, but beyond this restriction only incest rules apply" (1938:196). Among the Awa, women accompany the initiates to the stream and wash them (Newman and Boyd 1982:253). Among Bimin-Kuskusmin paramount female leaders are involved in male initiations (Poole 1982:116). Baruya women proudly turn their sons over for initiation: "Relations with the mother are more complicated. Until the age of nine a boy is dependent on her and on her affection. Then come the men to take him away, and she hands him over in a moving ceremony, gently pushing her son toward the young warriors who will carry him off to the world of men, beneath a hail of blows. All the women I have ever questioned after this ceremony have told me of their acquiescence and pride at watching their son going off to become a man, capable of protecting them and succoring them in their old age" (Godelier 1986:153).

Tairora mothers arm themselves with sticks to ritually attack the initiation party, dance and demonstrate when the youths are returning, and even perform simulated copulation at these times. "They [the men] regard the performance as proper and good, a wholly acceptable statement by the women, as mothers, of their pride in the ritual advancement of the children they have borne" (Watson 1983:263). Siane women bring ". . . abundant cooked food for their 'victorious' sons (the novices) to distribute" (Salisbury 1965:62). Women are involved in Sambia initiation rites as well: "The attitude of women about their sons is ambivalent. Women resist the separation. At the Yulami initiation below we will see the ceremonial wailing of the initiates' mothers opening the rituals. Later they aggressively reclaim their sons for the frog-feeding on the danceground. . . ." (Herdt 1987:114). Among the Hua ". . . postmenopausal women are initiated into the secret male society and take on the ritual status of male vulnerability. They become *kakora,* a term usually reserved for the initiated male who is, because of his purity, vulnerable to the pollution of others" (Meigs 1984:48). Women are clearly involved at least at some points during Ilahita Arapesh initiations: ". . . there is no attempt to deceive; the women are aware that they are simply costumed men who are taking their sons and brothers away to join the flying foxes. In the song exchange the women reply with a standardized lament—having certain ribald passages of its own—before following in a group after the youths" (Tuzin 1980:96). Among the Chambri, "Chambri women frequently invade a men's house during the initiation of young men and are at that time shown the secret flutes" (Errington and Gewertz 1987:157). Van Baal reports that "The Marind-anim constitute a curious exception in this part of New Guinea in admitting women to their rituals, an exception which is all the more remarkable because the position of the women is in no way superior to that of their less privileged sisters of the surrounding tribes" (1966:501). During Bedamini initiations, "While only men perform a *gosei,* women's part in a *gafoi* is pronounced. The audience is spatially divided according to sex, but all females gather in the male section of the longhouse. This is the only occasion they do so. The drums used are 'male' and 'female' as well" (Sorum 1982:46). Women were also involved among the Kukukuku (Blackwood 1978:130–31). Apparently women can be involved in all aspects of male ritual except the penis bleeding, which remains a male secret (Lewis 1980:182).

It would appear that "secret," "male" initiation rites are neither exclusively male nor completely secret.[18] While women were not privy to all the secrets they were quite likely aware of some or even many. In a previous publication I attempted to explain the secrecy in terms of male power over women: ". . . like all magic, if it is to be successful it must have an element of secrecy. But, conversely, if it is magically to insure male power in a political sense, it cannot be entirely secret. You cannot exercise power if no one is aware or concedes that you have it. This explains, I think, why some secrets are known, but not all the secrets. It also explains why women, even though they may know better, give gifts to the *nama* and take the ritual seriously—the paradox that fascinated Read. His Durkheimian explanation of the *nama* was predicated on the assumption that women knew the secrets but went along with the charade because they somehow must have sensed the power of society itself at work" (1974:19). Tuzin has recently offered a different explanation: ". . . At the latent level, iconically linked with the penis-cutting, meat-eating, flute-playing, and all the rest, lives the one meaning that men cannot admit to themselves and women can never be made to un-

[18]As it seems clear that women are virtually everywhere involved in "male cultism" in one form or another, and as the data on this is by no means extensive or clear, I believe Whitehead's interesting attempt to correlate women's participation in the cults with their "visible contribution to exchange" (or with "non-gendered crops" and certain lowland New Guinea groups) (1986a:281) is questionable and certainly requires much further work and thought. Mary Hawkins, for example, commenting on Andrew Strathern's interpretation of the *Amb Kor* cult which attempts to show the interdependence of men and women in ritual, makes the following statement: ". . . by defining males and females as interdependent and operating in harmony *amb kor* misrepresents relations of unequal power as relations of interdependence, giving validation to the continued male appropriation of female labour by constituting it not as appropriation but as interdependence" (1984:223).

derstand: that by nature it is *they* (the men) who are excluded from the ultimate condition of all living things, namely, the ability to generate offspring—or, in our usage, to procreate. The tricks, illusions, deviltry and pageantry of the rituals are indeed a 'pantomime,' the serious purpose of which the women would not understand, because, fundamentally, the men lack the language and self-insight to explain it to them" (1987:9).[19] This is another version of the womb-envy argument which I have already indicated I believe to be incorrect, and it does not speak directly to the question of women's involvement in the rites. Here again, it is possible to raise a question about the meaning of "secret." When various ethnographers report that the rites are a secret we take that to mean something that other people should not find out. But as Van Baal pointed out there is a more subtle meaning—the "sense of something shrouded in mystery, inaccessible to the profane, something about which no knowledge can be acquired except by the hard way of penetrating into its depth, like penetrating into the earth" (1966:931). It is possible that some if not all of the reports of secrecy refer to this latter type. Without knowing precisely what transpired in the conversations between anthropologists and their informants this would seem to be another open question. Van Baal makes another very insightful comment with respect to the secrecy: "It can be maintained that the secrecy observed is a means to protect the ritual procedure against ridicule, because, being a human effort to visualize the unfathomable, this procedure necessarily falls short of its purpose" (1966:931).[20]

[19]It must be pointed out here that it is simply not true that men are "excluded from the ultimate condition of all living things . . ." and that, indeed, it is only males who have the ability to generate offspring and thereby procreate.

[20]Luhrmann makes what I believe is a useful explanation of secrecy which is as relevant to New Guinea as elsewhere: "Secrecy is about control. It is about the individual possession of knowledge that others do not have, and from the psychological consequences of this priviledged possession follow its effects in magical practice. Secrecy elevates the value of the thing concealed. That which is hidden grows desirable and seems powerful, and magicians exploit this tendency to give their magic significance. They can use secrecy to conceal their

Herdt has argued that the secrecy of the men's cults allows men to be in a different category of "being" (ontology) from other members of the society which allows them to maintain their priviledged position. "The ontology of secrecy [sic], in Melanesian systems such as Baktaman, is a collective and culturally-constituted reality that proceeds in a direction opposite to our Western conception: it imposes an intentional code of differentiation in relation to some persons and entities, and solidarity with others, in order to make culture and nature conform to their respective ontological categories and appointed moral developmental pathways. Secrecy, in this sense, embodies a totemism of essential realities and natures, rooted literally in the body" (Biersack 1982; Herdt 1981) (1990a:367). Thus: "Contrary to Barth, I would rather agree with Baktaman men that those excluded from their secret collective are perceived and conceived as having a fundamentally different ontology and nature than those who are initiated" (1990a:367). Although my understanding of Bena Bena male ideas of being are severely limited, I believe it is probably true that they conceptualize themselves differently from women. Women, for example, are said to share a certain quality with animals which men do not have. I am not certain just what this quality is but it appears to have something to do with a kind of generalized carnality. Even so, in my limited discussions of this I did not have the impression that they meant to degrade women. It was treated, rather, as a simple matter-of-fact difference between men and women. In any case, even if men can be said to have a different state of being, they could still have a "communal cult performed by men" (Barth 1975) for the benefit of the entire society and not just themselves. I will return to this point later.[21]

---

magic from scepticism and to give themselves a context in which their own scepticism may be muted. In other words, secrecy alters the attitudes of both insider and outsider toward the thing concealed, and in magic insiders seem to use this mechanism to bolster their ill-supported faith in magic's value" (1989:161).

[21] Herdt insists that this cannot be: "Barth's (1975) study of Baktaman ritual is a good example

A problem similar to womb envy exists with respect to male initiation rites having to do with birthing practices. That is, it is often claimed or at least assumed that men are imitating women in childbirth and that the initiates are being reborn through males. Here again, however, as in the case of the couvade, there could be a misinterpretation. Broude has recently argued that if you see the couvade in its larger cultural context it does not constitute an imitation of women but is, rather, only one element in a larger magical complex: ". . . Thus, in societies that have generalized magical practices meant to reduce uncertainty when the outcome of a crucial event is unpredictable, men who in general play an active paternal role also incorporate into that role a set of magical couvade customs to ensure the welfare of their children" (Broude 1988:909).

Chernela, working with the Garifuna of Honduras, has more recently argued that "When indigenous classifications are considered, it is apparent that the couvade is a dramatization of maleness, not femaleness, and manifests opposition rather than equivalence between the genders" (1991:53). She goes on to make a point that I believe may be particularly germane to the New Guinea case as well:

> Indiscriminate cross-cultural generalization and the associated grouping of diverse behaviors into a single taxon belies a Western symbolic equivalency: (male) parental behavior before or at parturition is "female." Since reproduction is rendered exclusively female, a symbolic recognition of male as procreator indicates female likeness or equivalence. Thus Western writers, among them social scientists, find all such male parenting behavior a form of female imitation and several attribute its practice to cross-sex identity conflict. The widespread use of the concept of couvade, the variety of behaviors which it covers, and the paucity of explanation for these behaviors all demonstrate the need for closer review of fathers' ritual birth behaviors

---

of the miserly theory of secrecy, largely devoid of local ontology. Barth (1975:47–48) attempts to argue, ineffectively I think, that Baktaman have 'not a male cult but a communal cult performed by men' . . . . That is, he argues for the existence of a single 'society' (read ontology), which happens also to have a secret collective" (Herdt 1990a:366). I do not believe that ontology and society are one and the same.

where they occur (Chernela 1991:65).

I am suggesting that when New Guinea men performed rites that gave the appearance of birthing they were not necessarily imitating women in particular but were, rather, symbolically enacting a broader pattern of procreation and fertility in general. Thus, for example, among the Gururumba, when initiating girls, men led them through a hoop made of sugar cane. This could, of course, be interpreted as emerging from the vagina, but the Gururumba conceive of it as being like a butterfly emerging from its cocoon (Newman 1965:78). Similarly, Gimi males say they model their initiation rites upon the fledgling hornbill's emergence from its hole and they exhort the initiates to be "true men like the Birds of Paradise" (Gillison 1980:146). Ilahita Arapesh initiates are said to be flying foxes during their long period of seclusion in the forest and their initiation rites, like most others in New Guinea, are linked to the fertility of pigs as well as people (Tuzin 1980:114). In at least one of the Iatmul rites the initiates emerge through the mouth of a crocodile (Bateson 1932:437). Van Baal describes various Marind-anim rites as symbolic of birth but also argues that what is really being represented is the origin of man: "To put it in more concrete terms: the myth of the origin of man reflects what happens during the initiation rites; starting as a shapeless being, nescient and incapable of action, man is given his proper shape through the heat of the *mayo*-fire and through the activities of the *ndik*, the initiate, who moulds his body" (1966:549). Barth reports for the Baktaman that "the idiom of novices crawling between the legs of seniors seems *not* to be symbolic of rebirth" (1975:205).

The symbolism involved in many of the initiatory rituals is by no means easy to interpret. For example, Schwimmer writes as follows: "The Managalese and Omie of Oro Province, among many others, represent the womb by a trench dug in the ground and covered over, in which novices lie embryolike and from which they emerge in a simulation of birth. This 'sacred womb' is like a phallus; and it is contrived by men" (1984:277). One might well ask here why, if it is a phallus, is it a womb? Is it a womb because Schwimmer so interprets it or because the natives interpret it as such? It could, of course, be both. Similarly, is it Schwimmer who interprets this as a simulation of birth, the men themselves, or both? And, if it is a simulation of birth, is it simply an imitation of women giving birth or an imitation of procreative powers in general? Here is another case from the Gnau: ". . . Though the crouching boy being bled over, and the boy or girl being spat red all over, suggested new birth to me, the Gnau did not agree that the acts reminded them of this. They pointed out that the boy does not necessarily have to crouch between the legs of his mother's brother for this, but that it is easier for the blood to drip down on him like this" (Lewis 1980:182).

Buchbinder and Rappaport discuss a ceremony which might easily be interpreted as having to do with birthing but do not interpret it in that way:

> The sexual symbolism of the *rumbim* and the oven seems obvious, but we do not take the planting of *rumbim* in the oven to represent the procreative act in any simple sense. . . . The process of the natural world is the cycle of fertility, growth, and death, and the planting of *rumbim* and *amame* seems to represent an attempt by men to impose their own cultural order upon the bounties and dangers of the nature by which they are both sustained and threatened. If the oven is a representation of a vagina, it may signify not only that the bountifulness of the wild is an aspect of the wild's fecundity, but that fecundity itself is an aspect of the wild. This is to say that the planting of *amame*, itself a cultigen, around the oven which it eventually overruns is an attempt to capture for the cultivated the fecundity of the wild. Since the *amame* is explicitly planted for the benefit of women, domestic pigs, and gardens, it is to lash sociocultural ends onto natural processes, or to assimilate the processes of nature into those of society (1976:30–31).

Marilyn Strathern, speaking of Eastern Highlands initiation rites, says of this: "Yet it is not women as such that the men are so imitating: it is another version of themselves" (1988:245). Gell, in discussing the *ida* ceremony of the Umeda comments as follows: ". . . In *ida* the men, unaided by women, mount what constitutes a dramatic enactment of reproductive processes, a drama mounted for the benefit of female onlookers, stressing the male contribution to the cycle of regeneration. One cannot say that the men actually enact the female role in any explicit way: rather they show reproduction devoid of any female participation at all. This purely masculine creative enterprise is essentially 'cultural'—bio-social regeneration . . . is made synonymous with 'culturalization'; the 'natural' cassowaries are metamorphosed into the 'cultural' *ipele* bowmen as the price of their regeneration. It is as guardians of 'culture' in this sense that men participate, in *ida*, in the sphere of reproductive processes, otherwise the monopoly of women" (1975:277).

The *ida* ceremony analyzed by Gell is not a male initiation rite similar to the Bena or Sambia ones, but it does have similar elements. The link to fertility is overwhelming:

> These arguments taken together make me think that *ida* is a "fertility ritual" only in a very qualified sense; it is *about* fertility, but is not I think linked to a specific anxiety about sago in particular, or even about human fertility in an overt way. *Ida* cannot be considered a magical act with a precise goal in view, even though certain details of the ritual can be interpreted in this way. It reflects a generalized concern with natural and human fertility (perhaps it would be better to say "regeneration") which contains elements of anxiety, repression over representation and so forth, but is not, in the last resort, dominated by them. It is also a celebration of the normal, the processes of natural and social regeneration which are part and parcel of ongoing social existence, however much certain aspects of these processes may be repressed. . . . As a fertility ritual *ida* is an acting out of the processes of natural and social regeneration in such a way as to place those processes in a framework of symbolic categories. It is an act of participation in these processes; a dramatic performance which runs in parallel to the performances mounted by nature herself (Gell 1975:223).

It should be quite obvious at this point that the interpretations put forth by anthropologists are virtually all open to question. What one person interprets as a womb, for example, might be interpreted as a phallus by someone else. What one ethnographer sees as an imitation of menstruation might well be seen differently by another.[22] At what age children leave their mothers is not always clear, nor is it always clear just what fathers do with respect to childrearing. Indeed, in some cases, it is even questionable whether or not there are or were initiation rites. Of course it can be argued that initiation rites vary greatly from one place to the next in New Guinea, and it also seems to be the case that some groups simply did not have such rites. But whether all groups had initiations or not there are still some remarkable and very basic similarities in their beliefs and customs, particularly those having to do with semen, bone, and ancestors.

In some cases, of course, the symbolism of birth is so obvious it can hardly be questioned, as in this case from the Jale: ". . . Consider the manner in which the boy is pushed out of the men's house: his greased body lifted up by an elder, very often his father, emerges from the dark interior of the house through its narrow entrance. A linguistic analogy supports my interpretation of this movement as an act of parturition, as the boy's rebirth accomplished by his agnates" (Koch 1974a:408). Saulnier has a photograph in which as part of an Asmat "adoption" ceremony a number of men lie down facing the ground with women standing over them in a row with their legs apart. Two couples, presumably being adopted (or changing clan membership), crawl through this human tunnel (1963:40–47). In both of these cases it would seem indisputable that symbolic birthing or rebirthing is involved. But it is entirely possible that what is being enacted symbolically are changes in status or condition using an obvious analogy with actual physical birth. In any case, why does this necessarily imply some form of "envy?" Could it not be simply using birth as a symbol for fertility and life in some more cosmic sense?

[22] Again, see Lewis, 1980.

5

Semen and Bone

The attitudes of men toward women in Melanesia have, I think, been exaggerated in the literature. While it is true that everywhere women are regarded as in some ways inferior to men, it is vastly oversimplified and simply not true that "women are derogated and despised" and, as I have shown above, it is also not strictly true to say that "They are forbidden to enter the cult houses on pain of death," or that they are simply "beasts of burden" (Lidz and Lidz 1989:31). I believe what Marilyn Strathern says of Hageners may be true for others as well: "The Hagen denigration of domesticity is located within a specific evaluation; only with respect to activities that lead to prestige are things 'of the house' rubbish. That female concerns are thus denigrated does not touch on women's stature as social persons" (1988:89).

However, it does appear that—

> Even in procreation the woman is assigned a secondary part. She is merely a receptacle for the man's semen. Without a man, it is said, a woman is nothing; but the converse does not apply, for a man, as a member of the male sex, always, as it were, carries around with him the potentiality of fatherhood, requiring only the submissiveness of a woman to achieve expression. A closer spiritual tie is in consequence felt to exist between a father and his child than between a mother and her child. In childless marriages, too, the woman is always blamed (Read 1952:14).

The Baktaman theory is similar, ". . . the child springs from male semen as from a seed; it grows in the mother's belly and is nourished from her blood, which is why menstruation stops, but has none of her substance; it shares its substance only with the father and his clan, and can marry people from all other clans" (Barth 1975:77).

For the Gimi a man's semen alone forms the fetus (Glick 1963:100). "Having a child," one Gimi husband informed Gillison, "is something that comes from men. It doesn't come from women! Men give the child to women, women become pregnant and they must look after what men give them [the semen]" (1980:163). Gillison goes on to add, "Even a female child is symbolically male in the sense that it is wholly derived from the father or his ancestors" (1980:163).

> The Bedamini recognize that a child is conceived through sexual intercourse and insemination, but they believe that several acts of intercourse are necessary. Each time, a new part of the child is implanted by the male. The woman's womb is viewed as the temporary "house" of the child. Semen is thus regarded as an active substance with the potency to produce growth; but the mother's blood is also a necessary, complementary substance for a child's physical maturation. The strong bones, *gasa,* are thought to be inherited from the father, while the soft tissues, *hu,* are inherited from the mother. Strength and endurance are associated with masculinity, and softness and weakness with feminity (Sorum 1984:321-22).

"The Murik consider a pregnant woman to be a sort of custodial mother. They say she is just the *gai'iin,* the canoe or conveyance" (Barlow and Lipset 1990:35). Among the Kapauku, "The sperm fluid initiates the growth of the fetus in the mother's body and after the birth it increases the flow of milk" (Pospisil 1964:23). The Melpa say that both the father and mother bear the child although they distinguish between father's and mother's roles: "They distinguish between the father's initial work, i.e. his intercourse with the mother, and the mother's later work of carrying the child in her womb and giving birth to it. As a result of intercourse a man's semen surrounds a woman's menstrual blood and forms a package (*kum ronom*). Several acts of intercourse are required to make a child, since the function of the semen, according to Hageners, is to bind the menstrual blood so that it can no longer flow in its monthly cycle, and a considerable quantity of semen is needed to fix the blood in this way" (A. Strathern 1972:9).

Similarly, for the Paiela, semen is necessary to "bind the menstrual blood tightly enough to block its path," and "fertility is directly contrasted with menstrual infertility. This dichotomization of the woman's cycle," Biersack continues, "glorifies the male role in procreation. All other things being equal, the woman merely menstruates; she does not conceive. Despite the fact that it is the woman who bears the child, procreation is somehow construed as being male-dominated" (1984:129). Semen, for the Tairora, is

> first in the process of making a human being. . . . As a substance intrinsic to procreation, to be sure, maternal blood compares with semen in the making of a Northern Tairora child. It is inevitable and at least in that sense essential. But the indigenous view of semen is not ambivalent: there is no belief in the need for a subsequent ritual muting of its influence on the individual. The very idea might seem outrageous. Such an attribute scarcely makes maternal blood an appropriate basis on which to substantiate, as it were, the linkages of descent. Like semen, moreover, maternal blood is a simple substance, undifferentiated from one protogenetrix to another. It carries *human* information, so to speak, not an explicitly individual inheritance. In Northern Tairora society, furthermore, the progenetrix is an outsider to the sib or descent group to which her progeny will usually be assigned. As a powerful physical link to her, thus, maternal blood would tend to negate the main descent emphasis of Northern Tairora personnels (Watson 1983:257, 259–260).

Among the Waina-Sowanda peoples, "Because semen was considered the food of the unborn child, copulation was continued for the first four or five months of pregnancy," and the child is called his father's "egg" (Gell 1975:94). And again, "Semen is the food of the embryo: the child *is* his father's semen. . . ." (1975:249).[1] "For a Baruya, his wife's milk is none other than his sperm transformed into a substance to nurture his child; by giving her milk to young girls about to marry, a wife merely anticipates what the young bridegrooms are about to do, when they too [through oral sex] fortify their brides with their sperm" (Godelier 1986:57). And, according to Lloyd (as quoted by Feil), "A person's substance comes completely from his father, so only parallel paternal cousins are prohibited as spouses" (Feil 1987:144). Among Bimin-Kuskusmin, ". . . the semen of the father is said to form the 'fertile fluids' and breast milk. . . . (Poole 1975:10). For the Kaluli "Semen has a kind of magical quality that promotes physical growth and mental understanding" (Schieffelin 1976:124).

For Sambia "The womb is the container and transformer of semen. It changes the sperm into fetal tissue; primarily bone and skin, but also muscle and internal organs" (Herdt 1984:180). Among Kimam-Papuans, sperm ". . . is man's life-giving potency, powerful and beneficial. When, for instance, an epidemic strikes the village and causes many deaths, as often happens, promiscuous heterosexual intercourse involving as many people as possible is organized in the village to collect large amounts of semen (probably by coitus interruptus)" (Serpenti, in Herdt 1984:304). Similarly, "Women should assist in producing the male life-giving medicine: sperm, without which the transformation process from death to life is impossible" (1984:317). For the Usen Barok of Central New Ireland ". . . a man begets a woman's ability to conceive" (Wagner 1983:78).[2] Nilles wrote of the Kuman: "The physiological

---

1 But note that among the Yandapu Enga of the Western Highlands: "The Enga believe that a baby will die should the parents cohabit, because it may drink the father's war magic with its mother's milk. The father's semen is believed to be a potent source of his war magic, and it is said to mingle with the mother's milk within her body, thus constituting a grave danger to the suckling infant" (Gray 1982:77).

2 Apparently for the Daribi as well as for the Usen Barok the father is the significant figure with respect to the formation of a child; but Wagner's account is difficult to follow, as it is the difficulty of understanding conception beliefs themselves that he is attempting to

process of parenthood is but partially understood. The father only is held responsible for the begetting of offspring. He during intercourse plants the seed of the child into the woman's womb; the mother hatches and nourishes this till the child is weaned" (1950:30). Among Bimin-Kuskusmin:

> . . . both semen and fertile fluids are held to be male procreative contributions and, therefore, sacred, as opposed to the ordinary but polluting contributions of the mother. Thus, although menstrual blood is highly ambiguous and threatening, the fertile powers of women, which are of such ritual concern to men, are naturally male in origin. The male anatomy (and the male foods that sustain it)—in both men and women—is considered enduring, ideally invulnerable, and strong. It is associated with the most powerful of natural human essences (with the ambiguous exception of menstrual blood) and is intimately bound up with ritual efficacy (Poole 1981:128).

Even breast milk is regarded as a male contribution (1981:129). The Murik, too, deny the mother's role: "Thus the biological processes of conception, pregnancy, and birthing are condemned as unclean and therefore removed from the community. Thus the mother is not the 'true' mother but a vehicle for the fetus: the real mother is the 'bat mother.' . . . Admittedly siblings do share maternal 'blood' and paternal 'urine' which have been conjoined during coitus. But they are not of 'one womb' . . . since the womb is not part of the mother" (Lipset n.d.). Surely there is no compelling rationale here for the envy of either women or wombs!

One might observe here that even among the matrilineal Trobrianders, where women are claimed to give birth entirely without the aid of males, the woman serves primarily as a receptacle into which the spirit child is (somehow) placed and then nourished until birth (Malinowski 1922:146). And although the Trobrianders are said by Malinowski to be entirely

---

demonstrate in this paper. It does seem clear that semen is the crucial element in both cultures. In Daribi it is believed that men have only a little semen and must replenish it by eating meat. The Barok believe that semen is produced in the body by eating breadfruit, other fruits, and nuts (1983).

ignorant of the importance of semen, the newborns always represent former clanspersons. That is, the essence of what is being transmitted is an amorphous "ancestral spirit," which is no more female than male (Weiner 1976:39). And ". . . the only reason and real cause of every birth is spirit activity, are facts known to everybody and firmly believed by all" (Malinowski 1922:146).[3] The nearby Dobuans are said by Fortune to have similar beliefs about procreation but get angry with the Trobrianders because of their ignorance of the powers of semen (1932:239). Among the matrilineal Sabarl:

> . . . If "children" fall seriously ill, their "fathers" present them with a young coconut to make them "light" and healthy again. The soft green coconut flesh is said to represent bones that are not yet hard, not yet fully grown: the skeletal core of the child which is formed at conception by semen, and the lean/dry (*keve*) part of the body—the part that physically endures after death (Battaglia 1985:429).

This brings up two further questions that must be considered. Namely, what is it that comes either through or from females? And why does mother's brother so universally play such an important role? Among the Bena Bena, for example, just as a father cannot receive pay for his daughter, a mother's brother cannot receive pay for his sister's daughter. Although I was never told this, I believe the same explanation applies in both cases. Namely, a man cannot accept pay for his own semen (or, probably more correctly here, "vital force"). That is, what is being transmitted through the mother is not simply her female blood (or "essence") but her father's (and brother's) vital force. Nothing is passed down from mother's mother or mother's mother's mother, and so on, but something is transmitted that is essentially male. Thus when a Bena Bena man expels blood he is expelling the female element

[3] It must be made clear that there need be no necessary denigration of the female contribution here. That females incubate, nurture, and give birth can clearly be interpreted as being as important or more important than the male contribution (as Western Europeans are wont to do). But if one accepts the basic notion of the male contribution as primary, the female contribution and its importance is open to many different interpretations.

in favor of the male element which he gets through both his father and his mother. The Bena Bena term *bahalo* was translated for me at times as "male mother." He is supposed to be and usually is a nurturant figure just as is mother. I am not at all certain, however, just what "mother" means in this context. It seems obvious that when Bena Bena extend the term mother to all women in the clan old enough to be their mother it does not mean precisely what it means to Western Europeans. Similarly, the Awa do not distinguish mother's brother but refer to him as father (Loving 1974:115). The Enga say that ". . . it is purely accidental that a man's mother was born a woman, for if she had been a man, his mother's brother would have been his father, his cross-cousins, siblings" (Feil 1987:161). Given New Guinea beliefs about blood, semen, and bone, and their respective contributions to life, terms like mother and father seem to mean something entirely different to them than they do to us.[4]

Among the Iatmul, ". . . In the course of the ceremony the child is apparently ritually born from the belly of his mother's brother. This symbolism goes with a strong feeling that a maternal uncle is a kind and gentle relative and in initiation this gentleness is more practically expressed" (Bateson 1932:267). I do not believe womb envy has to be invoked here as an explanation for this. I believe, rather, it symbolizes the male contribution that comes through the mother, the continuity of the (essentially male) vital essence of the mother's clan and the link between mother's brother and sister's child. While it is true that the mother's brother wears a skirt during this ceremony it is also true that father's sister and elder brother's wife wear male ornaments. I do not believe this latter represents penis envy any more than I believe the former represents womb envy. Indeed, if the beliefs I have mentioned above truly exist in the minds of New Guineans I suspect those concepts are totally irrelevant.

---

4 Again, see Keesing (1985) for the importance of the problem of cultural translation.

The type of transmission process I have in mind might best be illustrated by the Bimin-Kuskusmin:

> . . . that patrilineage "agnatic blood," once transmitted through a female, remains "active" (*kwan*) in progressively weakened and less effective form for only three descending generations from that focal female, and is not transmitted into the fourth descending generation so reckoned. With the sole exception of the "agnatic blood" of his own patrilineage which is believed to remain undiminished over the span of generations through both ancestral and descendant males, the male procreative contribution of "agnatic blood" of the various aforementioned patrilineages, although infused in "semen" (*maiyoob gon*), is logically analogous to that of the female (Poole 1975:7).

Along these lines Whitehead has argued,

> . . . the purpose of semen transmission is not the reiteration of kin bonds, but the forging of bonds to and shared identity with males beyond the confines of the descent group. Affines or potential affines of the boy or his father, or the boy's father's ceremonial exchange partners are the men typically singled out as individual inseminators. Among certain Angan groups and also among the Kiwai of the south coast, semen from select "enemies" outside the community is even solicited. . . . While it is possible that semen of an initiate's agnatic kinsmen enters into the "pool" of semen that groups such as the Kiman and Marind-anim collect for besmearing their initiates or mixing with their food, agnatic (or cognatic) kin contributions have no salience as such. "Pooled" semen is after all precisely a form of the substance in which individual and kin identities are submerged into a unity, and in which only a single social essence remains in the foreground: maleness (1986:87).[5]

Even in the case of the matrilineal Trobrianders what is transmitted through females is not intrinsically female in nature but, rather,"*dala* substance." Weiner says of this:

> . . . Whereas, according to Trobriand belief, conception requires a spirit child (*waiwaia*) to enter a woman's body, this ancestor spirit is not conceptually identical to an ancestral founder of hamlet land. The former spirit is reincarnated from an ancestral being called *baloma*, while the latter is *tabu. Baloma* are amorphous figures of the past who through time are not

---

5 Along these lines it would not seem to matter whether the cult sacra are represented as ancestors or as a more abstract "generative force" (Whitehead 1986:89) as the underlying belief in either case has to do with maleness as opposed to anything else.

> remembered for activities in which they engaged as social persons. Only as *baloma* transmit *dala* substance in the form of a new child through its mother is the *dala* maintained. . . . Thus, the ahistorical (i.e. cosmic) cycling of *dala* through unmarked time, that is, *dala* "as it was in the beginning, is now, and ever shall be," is created and maintained by the blood which unites the reincarnation of *baloma*, woman, and child. In this sense, a person's "blood" remains pure and uncontaminated throughout his or her lifetime. No one can take away one's *dala* blood. As the Trobrianders say, "Same *dala*, same blood" (1976:39).

There is no indication that *dala* blood is female. Weiner also reports that she found no mention of any form of female ancestress and seems to believe Malinowski was mistaken on this point (1976:38).[6]

It must also be pointed out here that the symbolism in New Guinea initiation and fertility rites is overwhelmingly phallic. In the Bena Bena, for example, as for the Sambia, the sacred flutes are clearly phallic, Bena Bena dance decorations feature long black bird of paradise plumes that within the context of fertility ceremonies are also phallic, and some of the male dancers wear gigantic phalli decorated with small shells.

Arrows, another commonly accepted phallic symbol, are also often used on ceremonial occasions. Although one can interpret other items used by the Bena Bena in their various ceremonials as symbolically uterine (part of the dancing frames and strung bows, for example), I would argue that they are used mainly as props to highlight and thus emphasize the phallic ones. Allen, writing of the Big Nambas, says, "One might indeed describe much of Big Nambas culture as constituting a highly exaggerated celebration of male power, a

---

6 If Glass is correct in his recent reanalysis of the Trobriand materials it is clear that it is the male principle that is most important in procreation and continuity: "Topileta was androgynous, but his primary identity was male. On one level, fatherhood was banished to the supernatural realm and was locked into the process of reincarnation. Topileta was god, the ancestor spirit, but he was also part of every man and woman. . . . By an inversion, through the usurpation of the female reproductive organs, and despite the matrilineal formal dogma of 'no paternity,' it was the *male* principle that was supreme in Trobriand belief . . ." (1996:61-62).

feature no doubt itself generated by complex historical and environmental factors of which we are in almost total ignorance" (1984:93). He, like all other Melanesianists, concludes, however, that this male power is "directly modeled on the reproductive powers of women" (1984:119). Although I do not agree with all of Van Baal's interpretation here, he does give a picture of the overwhelmingly male emphasis involved:

> . . . The ultimate explanation of the dialectics might be found in the psychological consequence of a perfectly one-sided concentration on the power of the male sex in a phallic religion in which the female sex is denied an essential function and is accepted merely in an accessory and auxiliary role. The glorification of the phallus leads to the objectivation of this part of the male anatomy, thus degrading it from an integral part of the male self into a separate object. The inescapable consequence of the reification of the phallus is its separation from the human body; it results in castration and castration anxiety. Here, however, it is not an individual who morbidly concentrates on his sex, but a male community expressing its pride by erecting a symbolic phallus in the centre of the ceremonial grounds. The community of the males expresses its solidarity and its antagonism to the female sex in the glorification of a blood-stained magnified phallus and professes its contempt of the female sex by promiscuous acts of sodomy (1966:488).

Van Baal argues that men are powerless and that that is the great secret of the rites:

> Marind-anim religion is a phallic religion. All life derives from sperma and the phallus brings both life and death. . . . The phallus is the life-giving penis and the death-dealing *pahui,* the symbol used in commemorating the dead as well as the red-painted pole which is the centre of the *sosom* celebration. Everything derives from it and yet, the secret of the great cults is that the men must submit to the women, caught *in coitu,* powerless (1966:949).

Indeed, he argues that the frustration men feel over this is what causes their aggressiveness and thus their headhunting which, he claims, has no other motive (1966:949). It must be realized that this is Van Baal's interpretation based upon some of the Marind-anim myths, an interpretation that could well be incorrect.

Why, if men, and perhaps women as well, believe in male fertility, believe that it is semen which is responsible for life itself, believe, indeed, that it is semen which is responsible for insuring that women are fecund, need they be so concerned with the physical act of childbirth itself, an ability Bena Bena informants rather matter-of-factly pointed out is shared by dogs and pigs.[7] Furthermore, what does it mean to say that men are "powerless" and must "submit" to women? Surely it can be no secret to either men or women that it takes both sexes to produce offspring, except perhaps in the Trobriands (Malinowski 1922:155). This argument, like many others, simply *assumes* that men must somehow envy women and that they must envy them because they can physically give birth which men cannot.[8] As far as I know this argument rests completely on evidence involving pathological cases (Bettelheim 1954; Jacobson 1950). There is no evidence from anywhere, as far as I know, that ordinary "normal" adult males envy the female reproductive capacity.

In fact, the notion that it is females who are fertile rather than males may well be a purely Western European idea not at all shared by New Guineans. European ethnographers seem to be unable to accept this. Van Baal, for example, in spite of describing the absolutely overwhelming male emphasis in the rituals, makes the following statement:

> A nexus between head-hunting and sexual intercourse is, to all intents and purposes, utterly irrational. If it has a meaning—and, of course, it has one—it is the expression of the men's deep dissatisfaction with the effect of their sexual role, the subconscious awareness of their failure in the fertility process, on which their lives depended for meaning. Trying to achieve the unachievable, anger filled their hearts, and this anger drove them to acts of violence [headhunting] which could not solve

---

7 Along these lines it might be considered that apparently the Tauade gave the male genitals of their cannibalized enemies to their pregnant women "because it was believed they would give birth to strong sons" (Hides 1935:46).

8 T. Hays (1994) has suggested that if males were vitally concerned with the physical act of childbirth itself or had genuine womb envy one might expect them to be involved in childbirth, but they virtually never are.

> an inner, unsolvable problem (1984:164).

A few pages earlier he makes this rather clear cut statement:

> . . . His penis is no longer covered by a shell, but defiantly shown: drawn up with the prepuce pinched under the tightly fitting girdle, it suggests an erected penis, the proud image of male virility. It is not merely a sign that he is going to marry soon afterward; it is a reference to the fact that, among the Marind, *all fertility derives from the males, from their semen. Fertility is a major social value for them* (1984:136).[9]

The nexus he refers to is not utterly irrational to Melanesians.

Van Baal, like virtually all Melanesianists, is apparently unable to even conceive that the Marind-anim might truly believe that fertility is male. First he says, "The rites themselves give the answer. They are fertility rites, rites by which the men try to increase the fertility of their women, and to promote fertility in general. These rites are necessary because they claim that all fertility stems from semen and the exertions of the men." But then he continues, "It is a remarkable *pretense.* It reveals that the men are envious of the women and claim a greater share in the realization of fertility than is allotted to them by nature" 1984:162).[10] Van Baal, like all Western Europeans, believes that fertility is female. Wagner, when writing of Daribi, in spite of their explanation that an embryo is formed by semen "surrounding and 'holding' maternal blood in the uterus," (1983:76) goes on to describe males as "the second best sex" (1983:77).[11] Must New Guineans believe

[9] Emphasis is mine.

[10] Emphasis is mine.

[11] The only explanation offered by Wagner for why men are the second best sex is as follows: "But there is this crucial difference between them [men and women]. A woman always has enough *pagekamine*, or menstrual blood, in her body to form her part of the embryo—indeed the excess flows out of her body each month if not held there in conception. But a man's *agwa* [a system of tubes said to contain semen in men] contains a small and limited remainder of the semen released in his own conception. Unless this supply is augmented by the eating of meat, whose fats and juices flow into the *agwa* system from the throat, a man will have too little semen to conceive a child. . . .

"Thus a woman is sufficient for her ability to procreate, whereas a man, relying on the meat of feasts and prestations, is contingent. Women and pigs (or marsupials) are the essentials of childbearing, from a man's point of view, and society, from this point of view, may be seen

that also? What of the "extreme reverence accorded the penis and a belief in the extreme holiness of the male" recognized by Layard in the New Hebrides? (Schwimmer 1984:286).[12]

Among Bedamini: "The Bedamini males' theory of sexuality is given cosmic significance. It is believed that homosexual activities promote growth throughout nature, particularly in gardens, while excessive heterosexual activities lead to decay in nature as well as in social groups" (Sorum 1984:325). And again,

> The Bedamini recognize that a child is conceived through copulation and insemination, but consider several acts of intercourse to be necessary. Each time a new part of the child is implanted in the female. The woman's womb is conceived as the temporary 'house' of the child. Semen is thus regarded as an active substance with a potency for growth, but mother's blood is a necessary complementary substance for a child's physical maturation. The soul, *oeselibu,* is inherited in its totality from the father. A small child has no soul of its own, but partakes in that of the mother through suckling. The soul accumulates gradually in the child as it is weaned, and removed from the physical influence of its mother. Thus both men and women possess substances which will ensure growth, but growth can only be initiated by men as it is the semen, *ami,* that is planted in the womb (Sorum 1982:52).

---

as a kind of collective effort by the second best sex to corner its meat supply and keep things going" (1983:77).

If women form only part of the embryo they cannot be "sufficient" to have children on their own and, indeed, the Daribi, like so many other New Guineans, believe that semen is crucial because "The outer layer of the embryo, and the resulting human being, is thus formed by the father, whereas the blood and internal organs are provided by the mother" (1983:76).

Why the necessity to eat meat would make men second class escapes me, especially as meat is so highly valued in Melanesian cultures. And, finally, one cannot tell from Wagner's account whether it is he who attributes this status to men or the Daribi men themselves. The latter seems to me highly unlikely.

12"... we have to remember two facts. First of these is the high esteem in which the penis is held, as seen in the extreme reverence for the glans due to the operation which is itself a sacrifice. In the second place, the Big Nambas represent an extreme form of patrilineal culture which they have carried to a pitch exceeding all other New Hebrides tribes in the very low status which they accord to women. It would appear, therefore, that both circum incision and organised homosexuality are an expression of the extreme holiness of men over against women . . ." (Layard 1942:489).

"Milk, not blood," Marilyn Strathern insightfully observes, "is the cognized *female* version of *male* substance" (1988:216).[13] Even so, she apparently cannot avoid the implicit notion that males are simply imitating females: ". . . by masculinizing female attributes (womb, menstruation) men *imply* that the effective reproductive capacities of real women are male in origin" (1988:112).[14]

Biersack has pointed out that, "In Western biological theory, semen is not so glorified. Each substance, ovum and sperm, is held to be as necessary as the other. In Paiela 'conception' theory, however, male substance is singled out as the essential agent, transforming unbound blood into bound blood and infertility (menstruation) into fertility. This male bias stems, it seems to me, from the fact that it is the male and not the female who engineers the structurally prior arrangements and organizes sexual reproduction as a preliminary to social transformation" (1983:97). Andrew Strathern, when writing of female and male spirit cults, makes the following interesting statement: ". . . Thus, one theme of the cults is the question of which sex is responsible for fertility. In a society in which men stress their dominance they may claim that only they possess generative powers, a dogma, however, which they are likely to find is hard to maintain. As Lewis (1966:321), in a slightly different context, has put it: 'Here, of course, there is an obvious and vital contradiction, since whatever the jural position of women, it is they who are es-

---

[13]Emphases are mine.

[14]Emphasis is mine. I cannot subscribe to her argument that men (or women) are androgynous beings composed of both male and female elements (1988:213). I think it is more likely that male and female are fixed points of reference with males being the essentially fertile creatures women are thought to be by Western Europeans. Andrew Strathern has recently commented on this as well: ". . . Whether we argue that this reflects a transformation from an initially androgynous to a single-gendered state depends on the way the term *androgynous* is taken. Most specifically, the ideas involved have to do with 'weakening' and 'strengthening' influences, seen as the effect of gendered substances, and we might prefer to argue that it is these substances that are applied as an increment that can make a difference in the body of an initially 'sexed' but not 'gendered' initiate. Such an argument would make it unnecessary to invoke *androgyny*, a term with a physiological ring to it . . ." (1996:87).

sential to the perpetuation of life and of men'" (1970:574).

But it can well be argued, as the Gahuku-Gama apparently do, that it is indeed males and not females who are generative as it is only males who possess semen. This is a perfectly valid claim and no contradiction need be involved.

Yet another problem of interpretation becomes involved here: the distinction between that which is said to be "cultural" and that which is "natural." Anthony Forge, for example, has written of the "cultural creativity of men" versus the "natural creativity of women" (1966). Gell cites this and then says:

> It is as if the men, secretly resentful of the reproductive capacities of women, seek in their rituals, to compensate themselves for being biologically *de trop* by mounting elaborate cultural analogues of feminine reproductive activities. . . .

But he then goes on to say that,

> One cannot say that the men actually enact the female role in any explicit way: rather they show reproduction devoid of any female participation at all. This purely masculine creative enterprise is essentially "cultural" . . . (1975:277).

If the people involved in the rites do not distinguish that which is cultural from that which is natural why should they be "secretly resentful"? Furthermore, even if they do distinguish the two realms, why is that which is natural any more significant than that which is cultural? You see here again, I believe, the implicit assumption that fertility is basically female. But nowhere can females give birth without males so why is their contribution any more "natural" than that of males? Why is regeneration the "monopoly of women?" (Gell 1975:277).

There is one further important part of these belief systems that must be discussed here, beliefs having to do with bone and the relation of bone to semen.

The Bimin-Kuskusmin, for an initial example, clearly associate bone marrow with semen and also with ancestral spirit: ". . . the father's strong male blood is embedded in his semen, which is the biological medium of *finiik* spirit and the basis of the formation of heart, bone, and bone marrow" (Poole 1984:198).[15] And again: "First, male lineage agnates of a deceased man cut into his corpse, break large limb bones with a ritual stone axe, and consume morsels of bone marrow to ensure the safe and speedy passage of his *finiik* spirit to the ancestral underworld and to re-cycle his vital procreative and ritual strength within the lineage" (1984:208).

Apart from Poole's detailed discussion there is little information about New Guinea beliefs about marrow (although Andrew Strathern says bone marrow is "often" linked to sperm, 1996:108), but their beliefs about semen, bones, and skulls, cannot be ignored here. Remember that Bena Bena widows often carried the skulls of their deceased husbands and children were given finger bones to wear.[16] The Bena Bena were at one time cannibals and the brain of the deceased was consumed by members of the clan. The bones of the deceased were later returned to his subclan along with gifts of pork. Among the Baruya, people would wear the lower jawbone of a deceased spouse beneath their armpit (Godelier 1986:40). Among the Fore, women and children cannibalized the brains of deceased males (Lindenbaum 1979). Also, among the Eastern Highlanders Berndt worked with, bodies of deceased clansmen were cannibalized in the gardens and, in the interest of promoting fertility, their bones were buried there (1962:48).

> In Sambia imagination, individuals are born and die, but semen flows through them (along with blood) to recreate society. Individuals pass on. Growth as an aspect of these individuals dies with them. But strength persists: in the form of bones and skin tissue in offspring; in spirit familiars; in ghosts and spirits;

[15] For an excellent and detailed account of Bimin-Kuskusmin beliefs about bone, bone marrow, semen, and ancestral power see Poole's article, "Symbols of Substance: Bimin-Kuskusmin Models of Procreation, Death, and Personhood." (1984).

[16] There is a photograph taken by Hugo Bernatzik in the early 1930's which shows a Bena Bena woman from Kufagogo (Korofeigu) carrying her husband's skull. The caption claims she will carry it as long as she lives but I am certain this is an exaggeration. See *South Seas*, 1935, New York: Henry Holt and Company, illustration number 49. Also see *Headhunters of Papua* (Saulnier 1963:20).

and in the deceased's bones which after death may be used for sorcery (Herdt and Stoller 1990:83).

Siane girls, during the rites accompanying their first menstruation, are entreated to "Eat the powdered skulls of your ancestors, their arms and legs. This will bar the road to enemies. Do not forget this" (Salisbury 1965:73). The Kaluli lined the skulls of their enemies the length of their longhouses (E. L. Schieffelin 1976:13) and also preserved the bones of their own deceased (1976:159). Chambri believe that the child's bones are produced by semen (Errington and Gewertz 1987:160). Similarly, the Etoro believe bone and hair come from semen which contains not only "bone substance" but also "a life-growth force" (Kelly 1976:91).[17] The Gebusi say, when going somewhere, "as one bone we'll go" (Knauft 1985:63). Among the Paiela, those who own the land are said to own the "ground bone" and children are believed to get their bone from their fathers (Biersack 1984:121). The Wogeo keep packages containing the bones of famous ancestors in the men's club house and, Hogbin reports, "Some men even confessed to me that in extreme danger they had clutched the bones and prayed aloud to the souls for rescue" (1970:57). Among the Tauade, "The skull in particular was washed out with water introduced through the *foramen magnum*, with which the remains of the brain were flushed away. The children of the deceased are said to have drunk this water. Then

[17]The magical significance of hair is well known and it is often linked to semen and the genitals as well as to brain (Berg 1951; Leach 1958). Hair is employed by New Guineans in different rituals, very frequently when exchanged between sister's son and mother's brother as it is in the Bena Bena, the Waropen (Held 1957:144), the Mae Enga (Meggitt 1965:167), and I am certain among many many more Papua New Guineans. A man's wife cannot touch his hair, it is a prime ingredient for sorcery, and the like. Among the Baktaman, for example, hair is "the essence of potency and growth" (Barth 1975:78). In the Solomons hair is kept in relic cases along with bones (Ivens 1927:218). Among the Hua ". . . hair is a form of vital essence" (Meigs 1984:103). I am sure many more examples can be found. This is far too large a topic to attempt to deal with here but I believe the significance of exchanging hair between mother's brother and sister's son is most probably symbolic of the transmission of male substance rather than female. What you get *from* your mother is not the same as what you get *through* her lineage.

the skull was put in a string bag with the rest of his bones and dried over a fire" (Hallpike 1977:158).

Among the Abelam: ". . . In the case of a man, the skull, humerus and phalanges are exhumed by the women. The skull is painted with red ochre, and placed in the yam house of a son or brother. The humerus is used for divining theft, and the phalanges are mixed with herbs for yam magic" (Kaberry 1941a:362). According to Mead, the Arapesh used the bones of ". . . the gentle, wise, reliable man" for a variety of magical purposes (1935:142). These seemed to include hunting and gardening magic among other things:

> . . . The magical use of the bone dust from the preserved bones of the dead is also widespread. The Arapesh have a well-integrated pattern of chewing the bone of a dead male ancestor with a little ginger, as protective, hunting or gardening magic. Just recently, in the last four years, they have bought from their neighbors a method of divining which is based upon chewing the bone of a dead male ancestor who will later inspire the diviner while he is in a putative state of possession (Mead 1938:180).

The Iatmul ritually consumed a mixture containing the scrapings of ancestral bones and preserved the bones "as relics of . . . totemic ancestors" (Bateson 1932:427-28). Among the Gnau, ". . . men do eat scrapings from their own father's jawbones in various rites" (Lewis 1980:175). The Hua carried the bones of loved ones in packets around their necks (Meigs 1984:111). Among the Dugum Dani, where corpses are ordinarily cremated, a woman searches through the cold ashes picking out the remaining bones which are placed in a banana leaf and subsequently placed with other such relics in a special place behind the men's house (Heider 1970:156). Buchbinder and Rappaport report that for the Maring—

> . . . The treatment of the remains of married men whose wives survive them is more protracted. While the bones of their torsos and legs are interred soon after the *Ngimbai* in the pandanus groves in the lower portions of the territory, the bones of their arms, fingers, mandibles, and sometimes their skulls, remain in their widows' custody. Some wear the bones of the fingers and forearms as necklaces; the bones not worn are kept in net bags

> in the eaves of their houses. . . . After two years or so, during the final days of a pig festival (*Kaiko*), should one occur during the period of mourning, the bones are finally interred at the *raku*, the hallowed place at which the sub-clan offers pigs to its ancestors (1976:24).

The Foi maintained all bones of clansmen permanently in a special place (J. Weiner 1988:112). Deceased Gimi males were put on a platform to decompose:

> In two or three months, men calculate, decomposition was complete. Then they collected his bones, using sticks to lift the "powerful" remains in which the man's *auna* (personal life force) still resided, and placed them inside the hollow trunk of a hoop pine, inside a mountain cave and in other places in the forest associated with the regeneration of *kore* (collective male life force) (Gillison 1980:157).

Among the Kwoma, ". . . the skeleton is removed from the platform for final burial in the ground under the house. The clavicle, jaw bone, and femur of a man, however, are removed and distributed among the friends of the deceased" (Whiting and Reed 1938:216).[18] The Raiapu Enga are reputed to utilize "magic bundles of bones and leaves which are believed to be very old and are inherited patrilineally" (Feachem 1973:277).[19]

Among both Kimam and Marind-anim there are myths detailing how the coconut tree originally grew out of a dead man's head and the coconut used in a funeral is said to be a cut-off human head and the symbol of life (Serpenti 1965:212).[20] Among the Gnau of the Sepik River ". . . men keep some of their father's bones to scrape and eat them in certain rites, and so that their father's spirit will stay near watching over them" (Lewis 1975:38). The Ilahita Arapesh em-

[18]It is almost certainly the case that "friends" was used here for want of precise information as to who received the bones. It must surely be the case that friends included relatives as well.

[19]Feachem does not specify that these are human bones but it seems most likely they are.

[20]The myth of a coconut tree growing out of a skull occurs among the northern Mandek of New Ireland as well: "A part of the *euli* death feast rituals of the past was the exhumation of the skull of a deceased man being honored by the ceremonies. The skull was reburied in a specially prepared hole within a man's house enclosure, along with shell money, various foods, and a coconut. The coconut would subsequently sprout 'out of the head of a man,' thus reiterating the origin myth. The fruit of such trees was taboo to all females" (Clay 1975:82).

ploy the bones of the dead to help them erect their large spirit houses, ". . . a task which mere mortals could not hope to accomplish unaided" (Tuzin 1980:137). For the Garia, ". . . in the past before the substitution of inhumation for exposure of corpses, principals at pig exchanges used to cover with red ochre the skeletal remains—especially the skulls and jawbones—of the dead still kept in their houses, and either carry them on their persons or place them in prominent positions on the food poles set up for display" (Lawrence 1984:232). Daribi funeral rites involved cleaning and saving the bones of deceased clan members (Wagner 1972:148) as did those of the people around Lake Kutubu (Williams 1940:123).[21] The Waropen preserved and featured skulls in their death rituals (Held 1957:183).[22] Barth says of the Ok: "All Ok people seem to practice what may be characterized as a cult of ancestors, using skulls and bones of the deceased as sacred relics" (Barth 1987:3). There were elaborate ceremonies surrounding the skull in the Torres Straits (Haddon 1904:248). Although no further details are given, Nilles reports that the Kuman allowed the flesh to decay and then interred

[21]Indeed, Williams recorded a shaman's spell "which begins with a catalogue of the founder's bones—spine, neck-vertebrae, skull, lower jaw, shins, etc.—and it was made clear that these corresponded with the sticks and stones which would ostensibly be dragged out of the sufferer's body" 1940:57). Finger bones are also featured in male initiations as each of the initiates is given a string bag which, among other things, contains them (p.55).

[22]With respect to skulls it appears that in some parts of the New Hebrides and the Banks Islands (and perhaps elsewhere in that general area as well) corpses were buried with only their heads exposed to facilitate the removal of the skull (Layard 1942:532). At least some of the Solomon Islanders preserved the skulls, jawbones, and other relics of the deceased as well, often kept in specially carved "relic cases" (Ivens 1927:214). According to Codrington, the people of the Island of Ysabel kept the skulls of their chiefs and also hunted heads for them: "When a chief dies, they bury him so that his head is near the surface, and over it they keep a fire burning, so that they may take up the skull for preservation in the house of the man who succeeds to power. An expedition then starts to procure heads in honor of the deceased, now become a *tindadho* to be worshipped. Anyone not belonging to the place will be killed for the sake of his head, and the heads procured are arranged upon the beach, and believed to add *mana*, spiritual power, to the new *tindadho*. . . ." (1969:257). He also reports that skulls were hung up in other areas of the Solomons and the New Hebrides as well (1969:345). Among the Kwaio skulls are exhumed as sacred relics (Keesing 1982:64).

the bones (1950:39).[23] Among the Melpa, ". . . The father's *ndating* shows in the son's body and head hair, his genitals, and in his manly ability to make speeches and fight" (A. Strathern 1970:580). Among the Murik, "Until the 1930's, bones used were exhumed during mourning approximately six weeks after death. The *mwara* kin cleansed and washed them as a service to the ghost, which was later repaid by the Washing Feast" (Lipset n.d. 53).[24]

"Another way of expressing this is to say that he has his father's 'bone' (*ombil*)" (A. Strathern 1972:10). Similarly, among the Paiela, "Every ancestor is associated with a bounded territory whose 'bone' his descendents 'own'" (Biersack 1983:87).

Although the Trobrianders are not, strictly speaking, Papua New Guineans, their practices are interesting enough to record here:

> The excision of the bones and their subsequent use as relics is an act of piety; the process of detaching them from the putrifying corpse, a heavy, repugnant, and disgusting duty. The sons of the deceased are expected by custom to curb and conceal their disgust, and to suck some of the decaying matter when they are cleaning the bones. Speaking with virtuous pride they will say: "I have sucked the radius bone of my father; I had to go away and vomit; I came back and went on." After they have cleansed the bones, which is always done on the seashore, they return to the village, and the dead man's kinswomen ceremonially "wash their mouths" by giving them food and purify their hands with coconut oil. The bones are converted to various purposes, serviceable and ornamental: the skull is made into a lime pot to be used by the widow; the jaw-bone is turned into a neck ornament to hang on their breast; the radius, ulna, tibia, and some other bones are carved into lime spatulae to be used

---

23 Apparently among the Telefolmin bones are believed to be created entirely from the mother's menstrual blood (Barth 1987:14). This appears, again, to be an unusual case.

24 Lipset goes on here to say: ". . . The bones were not signs of agnatic substance which had been finally rid of maternal flesh, but simply objects of nurture (and emblems of taboo) to be looked after by the widow or widower 'like children.' After the Washing Feast, they were construed as sources of agency and protection, but not of fertility." Lipset's account of the Murik's beliefs about human nature, sexuality, death, and reproduction are far too complex to go into here, but I believe they could be interpreted differently.

with betel and areca nut (Malinowski 1922:133).

It may be of significance to note here that the exhumation and treatment of the bones is done by a man's *sons*, who keep some of the bones as "relics," and distribute others to their "relatives" [?] (1922:132).

Weiner also comments on this: "After the *sagali*, the skull is returned to the caretaker, usually the *father* or *sons* of the deceased. Often the skull is guarded in this way for ten or twenty years. Finally the skull is again decorated. Workers now carry the skull to the beach, placing it on a cliff overlooking the sea" (Weiner 1976:84).[25] The Dobuans keep the skull of the deceased and with it dance his spirit to *Bwebweso*, the abode of the dead on Normandy Island (Fortune 1932:277). Van Baal has given an extremely detailed account of Marind-anim headhunting and how the skulls are prepared and used in ritual. There is no doubt about the link to fertility: "New life sprouts from the dead coconut [used in ritual] as well as from the beheaded enemy. That the names of the victims are given to young children seems to hold the inference that somehow headhunting is believed to promote fertility and well-being, vague though this belief may be. They are, as it were, the fruits of the headhunt, the tangible proof of its salutary effect" (1966:754). The Marind-anim also exhume the skeletons of their deceased and employ the skulls in ritual (1966:773).

Consider also the well-known case of the Asmat:

> The ancient concept of maleness as a finitely limited substance that must be taken from others is well developed among the Asmat of Papua, an almost untouched tribe who were cannibals and headhunters until about 1954. But cannibalism was not the chief end of their headhunting, only a secondary adjunct to it: The getting of virility and of fertility are the real goals. To this end, the brains of enemy victims are eaten by the old men, soon to be ritual ancestor-spirits, and the decorated head of the enemy victim is placed in the groin of the adolescent initiate, soon to become a man. "For a considerable time the skull must

[25] Emphases are mine.

> rest between the thighs of the initiate, almost touching his genitals; thus there is thought to be a relationship between the skull and the genitals of the youngster, whose initiation marks his entry into manhood." The initiate not only absorbs the vitality of the headhunted victim but also takes on his name (La Barre 1984:36).[26]

Lattas has recently written on the question of gender relations in West New Britain and makes the following statement which perhaps sums up the situation for Papua New Guinea as well:

> Perhaps the ultimate generative image of the "true man" of exchange is the man who has bone in his penis: "If his penis has not got bone, he will not be able to pay back this something. If you have bone you will work what I have worked for you." The "working of bone" refers partly to the strenuous labor necessary for acquiring items of exchange such as shell money, pigs, and garden produce. Shell money is often referred to metaphorically both as bone and semen. Bones are seen as formed in the womb from semen; they are the basis of male strength. A man requires "bone" to establish large gardens for the giving of debts. "Bone" is also used as a metaphor to refer to something true or essential, to some defining characteristic. Whereas the female components of the body (flesh and blood) decompose quickly upon death, bones are recogized as being more permanent (traditionally they were dug up to participate in ceremonies). Through their semen men embody the bones of life, what is essential in it, and this they transpose into the "seminal" process of giving. They are engaged in the process of giving what is essential, what is corporeally permanent, and in doing so they essentialize and disseminate the process of giving. "This something is my semen and bone. Here is your shell money and pig. You now hold my bone, my strength has gone" (1990:93).

Battaglia has given an interesting account from the matrilineal Sabarl where gifts referred to as "bones" are given by

---

[26]The identification of trophy heads with both phallus and fertility has been reported from other parts of the world as well. Among the Iban of Borneo, for example, "At this culminating point of a head-hunting ritual then, trophy heads and the rice seed (*benih padi*), on the fertility of which the welfare of the Iban principally rests, are directly equated. Indeed, the trophy head, phallic and procreative, becomes a veritable fount of fertility—a most potent object which not only confers an undying prestige on the warrior who has procured it, but becomes, for his community, a source from which their sacred *padi* may draw an ever-continuing fecundity" (Freeman 1979:243). See also Hutton (1928) and Jensen (1974).

fathers' sisters' children (referred to as "fathers") to mothers' brothers' children (called "children"). She says of this: "'Bones,' then, refer to the artifacts of paternal nurture—the beginning and end of the physical person and the endowments from paternal kin. As a masculine, lean/dry component of the body, they also represent invulnerability to decay, relative at least to their feminine lean/dry counterpart: the flesh of the body produced by the mother's blood" (1985:430).

Although the association of bone with semen is extremely widespread it is apparently not universal. Among the Huli, for example, it is believed that a child's flesh originates from semen and its bones from menstrual blood (Glasse 1968:60). This is apparently the case for the Daribi as well: ". . . *Kawa* 'semen' forms the skin, muscle tissue, and external parts of the body, is contained in the network of *agwa bono* 'lymphatic vessels' and is transmitted by males. *Pagekamine* 'base, maternal blood' forms the bones, viscera, and internal organs of the body, is contained in the network of *kigibidi* 'blood vessels' and is transmitted by females" (Wagner 1980:426). Jorgenson reports that Telefolmin women claim that it is their womb blood that creates bones. This belief is apparently not shared by men but the issue is not entirely clear:

> . . . While it is indeed true that semen and vaginal fluids go to form the foetus, and that these are thoroughly mixed together in the process, this only accounts for the child's flesh and blood. My "mother" asked me, now, if I had wondered where the infant's *bones* came from, or if I knew why women ceased menstruating after they had conceived. . . . The answer is that the flesh and blood are formed equally by both parents, but it is the *mother alone* who provides the child's bones through the accumulation of her womb blood (1983a:61).

The Telefolmin otherwise resemble most other New Guineans in that they have male initiations, believe semen is necessary to form children, and use the bones of deceased persons in their religious rites. Assuming these ethnographers have correctly interpreted these beliefs they would seem to represent somewhat unusual cases.

The belief that semen originates in the brain and travels

down the spine to the penis is also very widespread throughout the world (La Barre 1984:3). It certainly occurs in New Guinea. Thus, we can find a Sambia informant stating that "Semen makes the infant, completely: bone, skin, brain [including the spinal column]. . . . One thing only—blood—your momma gives to you" (quoted in Herdt 1981:217). They also say "The semen organ is joined by 'feeder tubes' to the mouth, navel and penis" (1981:218). Among the Huli the spine is believed to be a conduit of semen from the head (A. Strathern 1996:125). Similarly the Baruya chew magical nuts to gain sperm and "The magic power filters down from the roots of their teeth to their penises" (Godelier 1986:38). Gillison, writing of the Gimi: ". . . During orgasm the *avuso* in his bones and head, the glutinous, light-colored stuff that constitutes his bone marrow, nasal mucous, gray matter, etc., flows into his penis and 'shoots' white *hato* [semen] into the woman. . . ." (1993:202). The Daribi believe the human body contains two networks of tubes that semen passes through after it is produced by the eating of meat (Wagner 1983:77). Is it at all surprising, then, to find the Hua stating that "semen is stored in the head and travels to the penis via the spinal column" (Meigs 1984:76), precisely the same error the otherwise informed Leonardo da Vinci made in one of his anatomical drawings (La Barre 1984:3)?[27] Interestingly, the skull is linked to birth by the Kwaio:

> The skull is an ideal symbolic vehicle for expressing the transition from the physical to the immaterial, from mortality to immortality, a process of death and rebirth. The skull physically survives for centuries, as a visible transformation of the known human individual. In size and shape, the skull lends itself to symbolically representing an infant; and exhumation

[27] This was a common belief for the early Greeks: "The final point here is that the head was seen as the seat of life in another, concrete sense as the vessel of the procreative seed or semen, transmitted to the male testes via the cerebrospinal column. . . . The association of head with semen also explains the form of representations of the god Hermes as a phallus with a head at the top. Hermes was generative power, also the 'giver of increase, wealth' . . ." (A. Strathern 1996:47).

> itself becomes an analogue of birth—birth from the earth of symbolic origins to which mortal remains have been returned (Keesing 1982:175).

While it is true that bones are of basic importance to the human body, and because of their relative permanence might obviously be chosen for human ritual purposes, these widespread, virtually universal, New Guinean beliefs about bone and their link to semen, males, and ancestors or ancestral substance simply cannot be coincidental. Given the incredible variation in New Guinea societies that anthropologists have reported this appears to me rather astounding. It would also seem to me to represent a belief system of great antiquity as well as perhaps the basic foundation upon which male dominance and the masculine ethos rests.

6

The Initiation Rites

Whatever the particular forms of exegesis, and assuming that the rites do not in fact create semen where it would not otherwise exist, strengthen males by removing "mothers' blood, or otherwise magically change youths into flying foxes, hornbills, or whatever, what might a reasonably detached outside observer conclude about the initiation rites and associated customs? That is, what do the initiation rites *do*? Let us leave the realm of exegesis for now and consider some of the more practical consequences that seem to be associated with the initiation rites. It appears to me that male initiation rites, as has often been emphasized, have to do primarily with fertility and continuity and are, thus, importantly religious in their orientation. Within this context four vital and related human concerns are emphasized: sexuality, enculturation, authority, and violence.

Pre-Oedipal may not be a very appropriate term if there is no subsequent Oedipal period. But if pre-Oedipal simply refers to the fact that an infant comes to love his mother "as a result of her feeding and looking after him" (Freud [1931] 1968:228), there can be little doubt that this occurs in the Bena Bena as well as everywhere else. One of the assumptions of the Whiting psychoanalytically based interpretation of the cause of male initiation rites is that the mother, being sexually frustrated during the long postpartum sex taboo, will act seductively toward her son and thereby receive at least some form of sexual gratification. As there is no detailed study of either childrearing or heterosexuality in the New Guinea Highlands, specifically how mothers treat their infants in this respect is not well known. One could argue that Bena Bena women, like men, feared sexual relations and engaged in them only infrequently and under duress. If this could be established it might be possible to then argue they were not sexually frustrated and therefore did not act seductively toward their sons. But as we do not truly know what ordinary marital sex was like for most Papua New Guineans, we are hardly in a position to answer this question.

The picture I have of marital sexual relations among the Bena Bena indicates that a man would visit his wife frequently when trying to conceive a child (the belief that repeated acts of intercourse were necessary is, as far as I know, virtually universal throughout New Guinea). Once a woman was known to be pregnant further sexual relations (supposedly) stopped. The couple would then abstain from sex, they reported, until the child cut its second tooth. The sex act took place in private, usually in the woman's house (although adulterous relations took place in the gardens or "bush"). There was said to be no foreplay. There are, however, reasons for questioning this description: (1) There clearly was foreplay involved in the courting ceremonies and we would have to presume this ceased entirely during marriage,[1] (2) there were obvious bonds of affection between at least some husbands and wives, (3) at least some men admit to breaking the rules of abstinence, (4) some men admitted to favoring one wife or sexual partner over others, and (5) love magic was employed, at least by males, to attract members of the opposite sex. This is consistent also with Herdt's claim that Sambia men are erotically

[1] There clearly was some form of foreplay involved in Sambia marital sex (Herdt and Stoller 1990).

aroused by observing children breast feeding and are "sex starved" before the postpartum taboo is lifted (1981:211). That they are actively interested in and enjoy sex is quite clear in Herdt and Stoller (1990).

Similarly, the Auyana acknowledge that abstinence from sex can be a hardship (Robbins 1982:111). Likewise, both Gadsup males and females are said to "seek sexual satisfactions and hope to find them in their marriage partners . . ." (Leininger 1966:169). Among the Huli "A man may take a second wife to gain a sexual partner while his first wife is feeding a child, a period of from two to three years when sexual intercourse is forbidden the nursing mother" (Glasse 1968:62). According to Berndt, in the Eastern Highlands,

> Through sexual activity a man justifies his status as a male, and the more he engages in this activity, the more highly are his strength and powers assessed (1962:129).

Also,

> There is a desire on the part of girls as well as boys to develop their sexual powers to the maximum through the stimulation of the conventional courtship meetings or in the permitted freedom during the premarital stage. But although this is to some extent channelized in marriage, the development of sexuality, along with other factors, apparently can find satisfaction only in extramarital liaisons of a spasmodic or permanent nature. There is a tendency to sexual excess . . . .

Indeed, according to Berndt, [marriage] "Partners are chosen and discarded largely according to the degree of sexual satisfaction attained . . ." (1962:127).

Although Maring men regard sexual intercourse as dangerous, according to Buchbinder and Rappaport, older Maring men can be openly lecherous and younger men are obviously interested in sex (1976:21). Barth, writing of the Baktaman, says: "Both sexes freely express mutual desire and a positive evaluation of intercourse" (1975:204). Kove women "practise love magic, and are often reported to initiate sexual advances and to request marriage" (Chowning 1987:142). The Mundugamor engage in passionate love affairs (Mead 1935:215). This is quite unlike the Mae Enga of the Western

Highlands who are reported to be particularly prudish and have sex with their wives only when begetting children (Meggitt 1964:210). A more extreme case is the Grand Valley Dani who are claimed to have a five-year postpartum sex taboo and be in general uninterested in sex (Heider 1976). Beatrice Blackwood observed that among at least some of the Kukukuku (nowadays Anga) peoples there was a lack of interest in sex:

> The conspicuous absence of plants used in connection with love magic, which made up so large a part of my collection from Bougainville, may be due partly to the greater secretiveness of the Kukukuku, and partly to my imperfect knowledge of the language. But it is also, I think, correlated with the fact that sexual interests play a minor part in the lives of these mountaineers, whose main concerns are food and fighting (1978:153).

The Etoro apparently taboo heterosexual intercourse for 295 days of the year (Feil 1987:177). It is here that one begins to see the genuinely paradoxical nature of male-female relations in the New Guinea Highlands.

In spite of the fears of menstrual blood, female pollution, and sorcery, in spite of the verbal proscriptions about the dangers of sex and associating with women, in spite of the stringent rituals that had to be followed by males, and in spite of some possible exceptions, the Bena Bena and most other Papua New Guineans clearly engaged in and apparently enjoyed sex. This can be seen, for example, in the fact that in spite of male fears of female involvement in sorcery, rape was a fairly common occurrence. Women did not walk alone outside clan boundaries because of the fear of being raped (it was common knowledge that a lone woman would surely be raped).

I am aware that in the United States it is frequently argued that rape has little, if anything, to do with sex per se, being, rather, an expression of dominance and violence. However, as the word for sexual intercourse in many Melanesian societies, including Bena Bena, is the verb "to hit," and as it is known that at least in some cases lovemaking can have a somewhat violent character, I am including it here as an essentially sexual act. Trobrianders' violent sexual behavior, for example, was described by Malinowski (1922). Lindenbaum reports for the Fore: "The language of intercourse is that of the battlefield or the hunt. Men 'fire their arrows' into a woman, and at first intercourse a husband may need to subdue a reluctant wife by biting her ear" (1976:56). Barlow and Lipset say of the Murik: "The expected outcome of a physical fight between a man and a woman (including married couples) is sexual intercourse and the Murik say that a woman who deliberately escalates a fight to the point of violence implicitly communicates her desire for sex" (1990:23).

Similarly, in an unusually detailed case, Herdt and Stoller report a woman claiming to have had an orgasm when having sex with her husband who had just taken her by capture (1990:183). Stoller has argued that at least some hostility is associated with all sexual acts (1979, 1985a). Among the Bumbita Arapesh: ". . . An atmosphere of sexual domination and conquest pervades men's descriptions of their sexual encounters with women prior to, and outside of, marriage. Men claim they most often dispense with foreplay, make no mention of the woman's sexual response, and use imagery emphasizing the sexual encounter as an aggressive act, an act of domination" (Leavitt 1991:898). For Gebusi: "'. . . Shooting one's bamboo' is an image commonly used by Gebusi men as a metaphor for their frustrated sexual intent. At one spirit seance, Gebusi young men actually shot arrows into the roof of the longhouse cooking section, as a graphic demonstration of how they would like to sexually 'penetrate' a reluctant spirit woman . . ." (Knauft 1986:264). Among Gimi: ". . . Women directly associate the first act of intercourse with the bride's being 'cut' and with her spouse's right to 'kill' her. . . . A man asserts his power to wound his wife, to make her bleed, as he prepares to submit to her dangerous sexuality . . ." (Gillison 1978:336).

"The Kamano associate sex with violence, as well as with danger and pleasure. It was quite usual for men to rape strangers casually encountered, errant wives and women of enemy villages. A single verb, to hit, is used for killing with weapons, killing by sorcery and rape, and I have heard it used also of rough but not unwelcome sexual advances by men. Victims of rape may become the wives of their attackers, and some adulterous unions are said to have begun in rape. . . . Sexual violence and deliberate infliction of pain are not judged incompatible with an enduring personal bond . . ." (Mandeville 1979:228). In the same area:

> . . . Through sexual activity a man justifies his status as a male; and the more he engages in this activity, the more highly are his strength and prowess assessed. His sexual relations with women are viewed as a kind of armed combat. It is conventional to force a woman, however willing, to the ground; in erotic play the pair burn or beat each other; in coitus a man uses his penis like an arrow, and the ejaculation is "shooting"; sexual intercourse is frequently referred to as fighting . . ." (Berndt 1962:129).

"The ordinary term for sexual intercourse in Melpa is *ronom*, the identical word which is used for physically striking an adversary. Accounts of raids are likely to tell how men went out . . . 'killing men, raping women, and slaughtering pigs,' where the same verb is used for each action" (A. Strathern 1972:247). The fact that men may be motivated by dominance does not mean they do not derive sexual pleasure from the act, or even necesssarily that women do not. For a very compelling argument about the relationship of sex to violence see Roscoe (1994). This is an obvious area for much further research.

That the Bena Bena apparently enjoyed sex can be seen in the formal and informal courting parties in which young men and women from different clans sang and courted all night long. The unmarried girls called out for partners, the couples lay down next to each other on beds of banana leaves, they "kissed"—this was also known in pidgin English as "turnim hed" (Meggitt 1964) and "carryleg" (Reay 1959)—the fire was allowed to die, and intercourse often resulted. Although Bena Bena informants usually claimed this was not supposed to happen it quite obviously did, not only in the Bena Bena but other areas as well (Berndt 1962, Langness 1969, Nilles 1950, Pospisil 1964, Read 1982, Reay 1959). There were also more informal courting sessions among the Bena Bena in which adolescent girls from one clan would approach other clans singing special songs to lure the young men out into the grass where courting would also take place.

Bena Bena and Siane are quite similar in this respect: ". . . From puberty to marriage, at about the age of sixteen, the girl is given great freedom and license, entertaining suitors at night and doing no work during the day. Girls of this age group often take over one of the women's houses as a clubhouse, sleeping and entertaining in it without supervision" (Salisbury, 1962:36). This also occured among at least some of the Eastern Highlanders with whom Berndt worked (1962:117). Among the Kuma:

> Women do not accept docilely a double standard of sexual morality. A wife does not approve of her husband's participation in courting ceremonies and extra-marital sexual relations with unmarried girls, though everyone else does. She herself is bound to the one husband, she is unable to participate in courting ceremonies, and her extra-marital relations (if they are discovered) count as adultery. This is in marked contrast with the licence accorded her before marriage, when she was free to summon men to "carryleg" and make love to her (Reay 1959:82).

Related here is the fact that unmarried adolescent girls do occasionally become pregnant, much to the consternation of their parents and guardians.

Similarly, adultery among the Bena Bena was by no means uncommon although the woman involved could be severely punished and the offending man would at very least be shot in the thigh with a special type of arrow kept by all adult males for just this purpose. Likewise, as there was an extended period of time between the appearance of a bride and her taking up conjugal relations with her husband, it sometimes happened that a new wife would engage in sex with her husband's brother or even his father before her own marriage was consummated. When this happened the woman was invariably blamed and returned to her own people and the bride-price refunded. As Read has indicated for the Gahuku-Gama, this possibility was one of the reasons the youths were urged to grow up quickly (1982:71).[2]

Even though women were said to be dangerous and polluting, men, especially the newly initiated youths, wore love magic to the pig exchanges and "sing-sings" specifically to attract women. If a youth could convince a woman from another clan to run away with him this was regarded as a positive conquest even though marriage virtually never resulted from these liasons. According to Koch, adultery was something to be expected of Jale men: "Whenever he [the initiate] appears to tire, his kinsmen rebuke him and say that if he keeps falling asleep he will never kill a man, never hunt a forest animal, and never copulate with other men's wives" (1974a:406). I assume this refers to the wives of nonclan members.

There were standards of beauty applied to both young men and women. Ideally, a woman should be slender with relatively light and clear skin, an aquiline nose, and breasts that stand up firmly. Although the young people of Bena Bena had little input into their arranged marriages they often attempted to convince their parents they should marry one person rather than another, their arguments being based not merely on personal preferences but also on standards of beauty and, presumably, sexual attraction. Whereas the parents looked for brides that would be good workers and politically suitable, the young people were more interested in those they met while courting and more "romantic" criteria. This is perfectly consistent with the Baruya case: ". . . But many Baruya hus-

---

2 Although he does not mention sex in this context, Newman reports that: "The first wife of 63 percent of the males in Miruma and the second wife of 40 percent ran away from her husband or was sent away because of her recalcitrance" (1965:26). There were five cases within recent memory of Bena Bena brides having sex with husbands' father or elder brother and being returned to their natal clan for that reason.

bands treat their wives affectionately; many youths fall desperately in love with a girl and eventually marry her; many girls end up marrying the men they wanted" (Godelier 1986:75). Similarly, ". . . As we have just shown, there is room, plenty of room, for tenderness, affection, and even passion among Baruya men and women. The exchange of women among men by no means precludes affection between husband and wife" (1986:158).

Among the Maring, ". . . despite the ideal of acquiescence to the marital plans of male agnates, elopement is the most frequent way in which marriages are contracted" (Buchbinder and Rappaport 1976:17). In the Waina-Sowanda area:

> Bachelors had very clear-cut ideas on their sexual role. While they remained averse to any institutionalized sexual relations, they remained amenable to fleeting encounters. They did not pursue women actively, but cultivated their appearance so that the women would be moved (they hoped) to pursue them. Sexual initiatives were supposed to be made by women. . . . There was a very marked category separation between copulation and reproduction. Bachelors had few reservations where the purely copulatory aspects of sexual relations were concered (copulation being part of the aggressive masculine stereotype, and an analogue of their occupation *par excellence,* hunting), while towards reproduction itself they maintained an attitude of disdainful prudishness . . . (Gell 1975:106).

Gillison has commented on the paradoxical nature of male/female relations as well:

> I emphasize the often wide gap between stated and practised norms because the following treatment of Gimi rituals may make it appear that men follow their own rules (or are constrained by their logic). If menstrual seclusion were honoured and if women were avoided to the degree men say is necessary, then women would have some autonomy. The effects of men's fears might give women the potential to dominate social and political as well as cosmological affairs. However, several women told me they often cannot convince their husbands or lovers to stay away from them while they are menstruating and uncomfortable (1980:153).

Watson, discussing the Tairora, suggests that with respect to sexual behavior their practice deviated from what they claimed should have been the case (Watson 1971:250). Similarly, Berndt reports cases of women accepting lovers in their seclusion huts (1965:89). Jealousy and resentment over sexual activity was not unknown:

> Resenting that their own opportunities for a variety of sexual experience have ceased, wives accuse husbands of being lazy and neglecting their work to go with unmarried girls. Not uncommonly, a neglected wife attacks an unmarried girl whom she has seen her husband petting in public. When this happens, she is repeating the pattern established in adolescence of aggression towards girls from other clans who stole her current lover.
>
> Many husbands and wives are mutually jealous and antagonistic, husbands accusing their wives of being deliberately childless and interested in other men. The pattern of pre-marital sexual behaviour, in which the girl takes the initiative and the man has to wait to be summoned, encourages men in their belief that women are by nature insatiable in their sexual appetites and promiscuous in their attachments (Reay 1959:82).

One could well argue here that it is not the reported *antagonism* between husbands and wives that needs explaining as much as it is the *affection* and/or the *desire for sex* that continues to exist *in spite of all the reported fears, threats, taboos, and sanctions.*

I can only conclude from the above that in spite of the beliefs about women and pollution the Bena Bena and many other Papua New Guineans were interested in and enjoyed sex.[3] They believed that women were intrinsically sexual, more so than men, and that they were prone to seduce men and engage in adultery. Whether Bena Bena women were sexually frustrated or not I am not certain. I do not believe they were unusually seductive toward their sons. But they *were* mothers. They did, of course, nurse their sons, clean them when they soiled themselves, picked them up and cuddled them when they cried, and were in general quite nurturant. As indicated earlier, however, mothers were not unique in this respect. Any

[3] It might also be pointed out here that in precontact times the Gururumba used female war captives as prostitutes and in the postcontact period there were voluntary prostitutes (Newman 1962:213).

given infant could be and was cared for and nurtured by any one of a number of females both older and younger as well as by adult males. What you have is a situation where boys spent most of their infancy in the care of females who individually and collectively nurtured them. But they also spent their early childhood being nurtured by both males and females.

Given the above, is it at all surprising that initiation rites in Melanesia have a great deal to do with the control of human sexuality? Indeed, this seems to be one of the most crucial elements in this ritual complex. Is it at all surprising that for some reason in the human species, like so many others, males are attracted to females and vice versa? This would seem to be a very basic fact of human life. Jung has expressed it very well:

> . . . Thus the whole nature of the human male presupposes woman, both physically and spiritually. His system is tuned in to woman from the start, just as it is prepared for a quite definite world where there is water, light, air, salt, carbohydrates, etc. The form of the world into which he is born is already inborn in him as a virtual image. Likewise parents, wife, children, birth and death are inborn in him as virtual images, as psychic aptitudes. These *a priori* categories have by nature a collective character; they are images of parents, wife, and children in general, and are not individual predestinations . . . (1972:188).

If this is not simply biological it is surely "precultural" in Spiro's use of that term (1979:101). But even if the need for females is experientially acquired, must it be acquired only from the experience with mother? Especially in situations in which there are multiple mothers and other caretakers? As far as I know there is no specific taboo on mother-son incest in the Bena Bena but it was certainly believed to be completely improper if not utterly ridiculous. Thus during male initiations the initiates are not instructed to abstain from sex with their mothers (yes, I know this is supposed to be totally unconscious), nor are they specifically warned about incest, but they are repeatedly and dramatically warned about violating other sexual rules, especially those regarding adultery. The literature is very consistent on this point:

> In the final sequence, the boys' old pubic aprons are dramatically cut with a machete by the elder Mugindanbu. The limp pubic coverings then become the focus of a castration threat aimed at the boys as a deadly warning against adultery. The flutes are played again for several minutes. Merumei then lectures and shouts at the boys: "When you are grown you cannot become sexually excited over the attractive wife of another man. You can touch your own wife, that is all right. The flute wants to kill you, for if you steal a woman, she will cry out like the flute, and her man will kill you. If you touch another man's wife you will die quickly . . . they will kill you. We are trying you out now for the time later when you might steal another man's wife. Then we would not just cut your grass sporran. If your penis rises and you want to steal a woman, we will cut it off." The elder cuts the old pubic covering midway between the abdomen and the genitals. "No one will help you, we will cut off your penis and kill you . . ." (Herdt 1982:63).

Similarly, among the Gahuku:

> This implies that men felt women *had* to be controlled, and I have no doubt this was the case; the palpable evidence of physical abuse (and it was not unusual) does more than merely imply it. But men also held the opinion that women were sexually unbridled, in contradistinction to the ideal sexually self-disciplined male. As supporting evidence they cited the fragility of virtually all of the marriages arranged for novices during their initiatiion into the *nama* cult. These rarely endured to the point of cohabitation about six years later, and men explained that the girls "outgrew" their teenage spouses and "could not wait." They attained sexual maturity earlier than men, and, moreover, the expression of their sexuality was not inhibited by any "biological" necessities to restrain it (except during the period between the birth and weaning of children). Penalties for adultery fell most heavily on them, and in such cases the stock defense of the proud, superior and "self-disciplined" male was that he was not responsible, that the woman had suborned him to do something clearly contrary to his own inclination and best interests. It hardly matters that the defence was often patently false, for it was the temptation of women *per se* that had to be resisted (Read 1982:71).

Among the Fore: "Women then, like red pandanus trees, are only partially tamed. The language of intercourse is that of the battlefield or the hunt. Men 'fire their arrows' into a woman, and at first intercourse a husband may need to subdue a reluctant wife by biting her ear. A truly defiant wife is brought under control by disciplinary intercourse, the husband and all the men of his 'line' copulating with her in sequence. Indeed, rape seems to have been a frequent hazard for a traveling woman, whose husband might be chased away while the men of the parish territory through which they journey ravage her in the bush. This pleasurable experience is described by men as 'eating wild mushrooms'" (Lindenbaum 1976:56).

In Awa:

> "Now hear this other talk." A man dressed as a young girl enters the men's house, followed by a man who makes advances to "her." He pulls aside her grass skirt and pushes her to the ground: with erect penis he mounts her and pretends to copulate. From the doorway of the house the "girl's husband" watches: he draws his bow. The young man sees him and jumps up, grabbing his weapons: the girl tries to escape, and the two men fight. They leave the house. The warrior leader continues to admonish the novices. "If the wife of another man comes to you, resist her. Do not hold women when you are in the garden. If you meet a young woman, do not look at her face; if you look at her and she looks at you, then you will copulate. If you do this, something will come up all over your skin, your body will be spoilt. Hear what we say."

"Following this instruction, the initiates are taken into the men's house, where they are further lectured about the social consequences of marital infidelity. In the men's house they are shown a display of bows, arrows, axes, and fighting sticks. These, they are told, are the instruments of reprisal which will be used against them by enraged husbands should they be discovered seducing other men's wives. The consequences of such a transgression are not only social, however, and the initiates are told that if they have sexual intercourse with another woman and then with their wives, the 'fluids of these two vaginas will strike one another inside you,' causing illness or even death" (Newman and Boyd 1982:277).

". . . In all the lessons in morality that the Baruya give to their young boys and girls in the course of initiation ceremonies are the most dreadful threats of death for anyone who strays into adultery" (Godelier 1986:27).

Even Sambia homosexuality is linked to the theme of adultery: "If you promiscuously 'play around' [with prohibited categories of boys], when you become a *nupos* [married man] then you'll want to adulterously copulate with all of the women. With some enemy boys, only with them you can fornicate. [Tali]" (quoted in Herdt 1981:238).

Buchbinder and Rappaport report for the Maring: "It seems to be clear that it is the sexuality of females that is dangerous to men. While this sexuality is most strongly concentrated in the vagina, it is not confined there. Women are saturated with it, and it may spread contagiously to anything with which they come into contact, most notably their clothing, the food they prepare, and the fires over which they cook" (1976:22).

Among the Etoro, women and witches are identified with each other because of their unregulated sexuality: ". . . The identification of woman and witch therefore refers in only a restricted sense to an inherent quality of womanhood while being fully applicable to the potential characteristics of aggressive and demanding femininity and unregulated feminine sexuality" (Kelly 1976:49). Among Kimam-Papuans "Female sexuality is potentially dangerous for men and for society . . ." (Serpenti, quoted in Herdt 1984:294).

The Mae Enga have bachelor cults whose ritual activities "are directed primarily toward protection from female pollution. . . ." (Meggitt 1977:63) which, among other things, apparently turns the young men into "prudes" (Meggitt 1964).

The situation in some New Guinea Highlands groups cannot have been much different from that described by Knauft for the lowlands Gebusi:

> . . . The problem of illicit heterosexuality is in fact quite great in Gebusi society. Adultery and its suspicion are major sources of domestic conflict. The problem is especially great since young bachelors must wait for initiation and subsequent marital opportunity until they are 17–25 years of age. Of 21 bachelors ready for initiation and marriage in three communities, fully one third (7) were known to have committed either adultery or have had premarital sex. In one community, initiation plans

> were canceled by the married men due to the amorous activities of the novices; the young men were forced to move to another community, where they waited until an initiation there eventually took place (1986:263).

Sex was a problem for the Kapauku as well: "'The Kapauku women are more sexual than men,' claimed one of my male informants. 'They even ask you for intercourse. They are never satisfied with their husbands. They look for other men. They commit adultery and thus cause most of the wars in which men get killed . . . All women are bad . . .'" (Pospisil 1964:46). Among the Waina-Sowanda, "Adultery is the ultimate motive of sorcery, and sorcery is, for Umedas, the explanation of death" (Gell 1975:111). For the Sambia, ". . . sexual impulses leading to adultery are a tremendous social problem in Sambia society" (Herdt and Stoller 1990:72).

It would seem obvious to me that one of the primary reasons for the existence and persistence of Bena Bena (and other) male initiation rites has to do with the control of human sexuality, especially the sexuality of young males, but also to some extent with the presumed or real sexuality of females. Sambia attitudes toward wives are probably not much different from those of most New Guineans: "Why are men therefore persuaded that women become sexually aggressive as they mature? This appears paradoxical, but is not so experienced by Sambia. Men sense that women's behavior is basically deceptive. Behind a woman's mask of reticence, men are convinced, lies an imperious contradiction. Women are not really prudish, they are priggish and wanton. Women only seem to be shy; they are, at heart, not chaste but repressed. Sambia men presume that their *wives* are lascivious harlots who, when at last unleashed, develop insatiable erotic appetites" (Herdt 1981:187).

Similarly, among the Fore: "Women's sexuality is the dangerous 'wild' which men must bring under control. Indeed, much of the ritual of Fore initiation involves males playing on sacred flutes (symbolic penises) which they tell women and uninitiated youths are voices of *kabuwei*, literally 'wild women,' a word that by 1970 had also come to mean a female prostitute" (Lindenbaum 1976:56). Interestingly, even in the few accounts we have of female initiation rites, the same emphasis occurs: ". . . The only exegesis I was offered about why [Ndu] *wala* spectacles embodied intercourse, however, was that they enjoined initiates against promiscuous behavior that might create jealously and strife within their husbands' subclan . . ." (Roscoe 1995:76). Similarly, among the "Babae" (a pseudonym), the rites are said to "domesticate" female sexuality (Fergie 1995:127).

The natural affinity of men for women and vice versa, springing from basic biological roots and subsequently encouraged by the early nurturance of children by females must lead males to actively desire female companionship and sex. During the precontact hostilities in New Guinea groups of related males could scarcely have allowed themselves to be divided over women, especially women who were believed to be overly sexual, seductive, and, as members of other groups, potentially dangerous. This is not merely a question of men envying the female capacity for bearing children and attempting to control procreation as such, but, more importantly, at least for social harmony, to control the basic sexual desires of both men and women which might otherwise have run rampant. It is the responsibility of adult males to enforce compliance: "It [red pandanus] is clearly a symbol of female blood, and the edict that it should not be eaten by unmarried men is a metaphor for the sexual restraint they should observe at this age, and of the political power of adult men to control the sexuality of others" (Lindenbaum 1976:55).

Tuzin has perhaps described the situation better than most:

> Women are the bane of a peaceful society, and as long as men never compromise their masculine unity, they will hold the secret to a paradisiacal world devoid of women and full of life's pleasures. Indeed, in this Elysium women are not required to produce babies, for men will have taken over this role as well—as symbolized in the curious baby presentation staged before the boys leave for the forest. A man's supreme loyalty must therefore be given to his sex group and to the important secrets they

> guard. No devotion to family may override this, and a man must be prepared to sacrifice—if necesssary, by his own hand—his mother, wife or child at the behest of the Tambaran. The discipline is harsh and exacting, but in the ideology of the cult humankind depends on it (1980:106).

The Karavarans are quite explicit in their beliefs about the disruptive nature of females:

> Women, thus, are dangerous because they undermine both the social and the conceptual order: they cause men to behave in a disorderly way and in so doing attack the very concept of order itself. Men deal with this danger in several ways. One of these is most apparent in the ritual surrounding the construction of the male dukduk, during which the men seclude themselves at the taraiu. By ignoring the existence of women, the men can surmount their divisive power and create male solidarity. Another alternative employed during ritual is to domesticate female sexuality by defining women with reference to their childbearing capacity rather than with reference to their sexual desirability. . . . A third alternative concerns the use of a preparation called *polo* [a coconut oil mixture].
>
> Polo has perhaps the most complex meaning of these alternatives: it is the most realistic of them in the sense that it contends with the full ambivalence felt concerning relations between men and women. Men cannot do without women: society needs their children . . . and men, moreover, cannot fully control their own sexual desires. On the other hand, men fight over women. Women are not only essential but dangerous . . . (Errington 1974:63).

Murik attempts to deal with the problem of sexuality have been described by Meeker, Barlow, and Lipset: "In what follows we shall see that the warrior identity is expressed by rituals of sexuality. These rituals affirm that men have the power: (1) to renounce the sexuality of women; (2) to possess sexually for oneself women who rightfully belong to other men; and (3) to surrender women who rightfully belong to oneself to be possessed sexually by other men. In other words, these sexual rituals affirm men's ability to triumph over their scruples about women's sexuality" (1986:57).

It would appear that New Guinea cultures, although all deal with the basic problem of human sexuality, have developed similar but somewhat different means for doing so. The contrast between Bena Bena, Sambia, the Trobriands, and the Mae Enga is an obvious example. Bena Bena male initiates are secluded from women only for a relatively short period of time after which it is only their new wives they must (and do) avoid. But, although they cannot cohabit with their wives, they do participate in culturally sanctioned heterosexual courting parties which allow them considerable freedom for the expression of their sexual drives. Further, the possibility of having more than one wife allows them to continue the same pattern of extramarital affairs until such time as they are too old or uninterested to do so. As noted previously, this is the same pattern that prevails among the Siane, Kuma, and many other Highlanders.

The Sambia pattern is much different. Here the young boys and the adolescent initiates are secluded and kept from women for years. In this situation one might well argue for the same necessity for male homosexuality one finds in prison populations. Indeed, among the Gebusi, who also practice male homosexuality, such behavior is jokingly acknowledged to be simply a necessary substitute for heterosexuality (Knauft 1986:268). In the Sambia case homosexuality is apparently more specifically culturally sanctioned, even demanded, and surrounded by a complex of religious as well as other beliefs. Even so, it seems reasonable to believe that the Sambia also understand that adolescent homosexuality is a substitute for a more potentially dangerous heterosexuality. For example, Herdt says of castration threats during initiation: "By this act, not only is homosexual fellatio enjoined, but premarital heterosexual activities are tabooed and condemned" (Herdt 1982:63).

The Mae Enga, of course, according to Meggitt have the bachelor cults which effectively keep the young men free of female contact and pollution but apparently turn them into the most prudish of New Guineans.[4]

4 The unbridled adolescent and even younger sexual behavior of the Trobriand Islanders was

The Bena Bena, Sambia, and Mae Enga, like all other cultures, have developed specific techniques for controlling human sexuality, sexuality that could in their precarious circumstances threaten their very existence. The sexual drives of young men must be controlled and, similarly, as women are often regarded as being both licentious and irresponsible, the prescriptions and proscriptions are also often aimed at them as well. This is true regardless of the fact that men may be merely projecting their own sexual proclivities on innocent females, perhaps a doubtful assumption in view of the overall cultural context.

It is also probably impossible to understand either the origin or persistence of male initiation rites without considering the nature of leadership and authority in the highly egalitarian societies of Melanesia. The Bena Bena, like most of the others, had a "great man" system (Godelier 1986) in which certain men, because of skill in warfare, oratory, exchange, magical ability, or force of personality were recognized as leaders and therefore endowed, at least in some contexts, with more influence than ordinary men.[5] These "men with a name" could gain considerable fame and reputation even outside of their own group, but even so, did not hold public office as such and possessed virtually no institutionalized or formally sanctioned authority over any other individual person. While a given great man like Matato, made famous by Watson (1971), might be able to influence or command the behavior of other men through the force of his personality or the threat of physical violence, ultimately people cooperated or complied only out of personal choice. Even an exceptionally "strong"

---

well described by Malinowski (1922) and is still another solution to the ubiquitous problem of human sexuality.

5 I have elected to follow Godelier here and use the term "great men" rather than "big men" as I think it more precisely defines the status of leaders in the Bena Bena. However, the case in the Bena Bena seems to me to be more a compromise between these two definitions. Exchange is quite important in becoming a great man but would not, by itself, allow an individual to achieve that status. But see Feil (1987) for distinctions between "big men," "great men," and "despots."

man like Matato could be ambushed or killed by others if he abused his reputation or was overly careless. Godelier has written of how even a great warrior can be given over to the enemy for abusing his position:

> So what is an enemy if you can ask him to help rid you of your friends or your brothers, enemies whose great warriors are so feared, and against whom one sends one's own great men? Even these bulwarks and pillars of the tribe's survival are liable to be betrayed by their own people. This kind of betrayal throws a harsh light on the internal mechanisms of political life and power in classless societies. For the warrior delivered up to the enemy is one who has misused his glory and prestige, one who has become a despot, subjecting members of his tribe to his own arbitrary violence (1989:178).[6]

Thus, ". . . A leader remains a leader only for so long as he can successfully dominate others, either through his ability to help them or maintain their respect. If he fails in an undertaking his followers are quick to shift their loyalties to others. There are always competitors for power and influence. In so far as leaders do not control land or water supplies, or other natural resources, cannot call on supernatural sanctions to back up their authority, do not significantly regulate labor or subsistence, and have little in the way of special skills or knowledge, their followers are always comparatively few" (Langness 1972:927).

Given this informal type of leadership, as Watson so insightfully argued (1971), there is a paradox built into the egalitarian systems of New Guinea. That is, the emphasis on individuality, especially as expressed in male dominance and aggression, is basically incompatible with the egalitarian ethic. Thus, though in principle there should be reciprocity and equality, in practice the big man system is vulnerable to despotism. But as men with the unusual power of Matato are infrequent, and as their power cannot be inherited by others, the community only suffers despots temporarily. And, as they desperately needed such individuals in the ongoing raiding and warfare,

---

6 Also see P. Brown (1963) on despots.

the acts of despots had to be endured. Watson described the situation very well:

> . . . if the overt and personal use of power is contrary to a Tairora ethic of equality, what is to be said of a hypothetical situation in which no men of a community at all evince strength in the forms recognized by the Tairora? To say nothing of its effect on the politico-military standing of the territory these men defend, their mildness would be counter to the ideals of masculine strength and aggressiveness. In matching one value, it seems, the other is contradicted (1971:272).

In the context of the pre-European contact New Guinea communities *had to have* such individuals and thus:

> To this end boys will be frightened, cut, beaten, bled, sweated, purged, anointed, and fed pork, salt, and special herbs in the course of growing up and being initiated. Impressive and secret physical measure for men, such as nose-bleeding and cane-swallowing, will be invoked to promote their masculinity and aggressiveness (1971:269).

Not all men, of course, succeeded in fulfilling the cultural ideal for strength and warriorhood. Not all became "men with a name." As is true everywhere, some men led and some followed. Great men, by and large, played much more significant roles during raids, exchanges, and other rituals than in any day-to-day capacity. All adult males, just like great men, did pretty much what they chose to do until someone was strong enough to stop them. In fact, to a lesser extent perhaps, this was true of women and children as well.

Great men in the Bena Bena, as well as elsewhere in New Guinea, had to achieve that status by demonstrating that in some important respect they were better than other men. Success in war and the ability to physically dominate others was perhaps the most common way to become a *gipina*, a "man with a name." Success in gardening and pig raising also allowed a man to become widely known as this enabled one to participate in the various ritual exchanges and to aid others with bride-prices, death payments, and so on. Unlike the Baruya case, where the status of "great warrior" was apparently clearly distinguished from that of "great shaman" or "cassowary hunter" (Godelier 1986), in the Bena Bena case warriorhood and gardening most usually went together. That is, a successful warrior was more likely to attract more wives, as well as followers, which in turn allowed him to have larger gardens, more pigs, and so on. As far as I know there were no men who stayed home and became famous merely through their horticultural skills.

Again, the Bena Bena were very similar to Auyana in this respect:

> Contempt was also shown for those who were continually arguing for peace. They were usually referred to as 'garden men,' which had three connotations: (1) they were frequently in their garden when actual fighting broke out and only managed to arrive at the fight when it was nearing completion; (2) they were like women, as gardening was primarily a woman's task; (3) they were more concerned with food and pigs than they were with getting revenge and frightening others, as fighting would at least interrupt normal gardening and husbandry activities and might result in pigs being killed, gardens torn up, and houses burned. I suggest that considerable contempt was reserved for garden men because the above alternatives were precisely the ones which tempted all men to cease fighting (Robbins 1982:190).

Among the Bena Bena a man who was merely recognized as a great fighter but did not participate in exchanges or have ritual knowledge, would also probably not become a *gipina.* To be a truly great man one had to know how to perform various rituals and have the ability to organize people for both ritual and warfare. Thus they also had to know the group's history and the meaning of ritual objects and have oratorical skills beyond the ordinary.

The grassland-dwelling Bena Bena did not hunt cassowaries (or much of anything else) and although there were shamans they were few and were known only for their specialty of curing. That is, one could not become a man with a name simply by being a successful shaman. Warriorhood was by far the most important element in becoming a famous man, but most warriors were also, with the help of their wives and followers, successful gardeners and pig breeders. As Watson pointed out for the Tairora (1971:269), New Guinea societies had to have such leaders if they were to survive in their milieu of frequent raiding and warfare. It was during male initiations that such leaders began to emerge. The youths were carefully watched to see how well they stood up to the beatings and other physical abuses. It appears to have been assumed that the eldest boy in the age grade would, all other things being equal, be the leader of his age mates. But the Bena Bena clearly recognized there would be exceptions and they watched the boys for signs of leadership. In small groups like Bena Bena clans it did not take long before everyone recognized who the dominant individuals were. They appreciated talent as it expressed itself in gardening as well as fighting but it was the latter that was most important. Those youths who rose above their peers did so by demonstrating their fighting prowess but also by showing greater interest in the rituals, the group history, and even the more mundane facts of life such as proper butchering and cooking techniqes and so on. In short, they began to know more than others and in this way would eventually take over the management of group affairs, including the leadership of raiding parties. They would also be in the forefront of the warriors taking part in the more formal battles that frequently took place. They would gain a "name" because they stood out and other groups would come to recognize their superiority. Similarly, as their names would be more often called out than others during the massive exchanges of pork, their status was constantly being reinforced.

Men with a name were indeed the bulwarks of their communities, but even so they did not possess formal authority or public office as such. No one *had to* follow their directions but most people did so as it was ordinarily in their interest to do so. Great men could intervene, for example, in intraclan disputes. If two or more members of a clan or subclan were fighting or there was otherwise bad blood between them a great man might kill and cook a pig, invite the disputants to a feast, and suggest that they resolve their differences. If all parties accepted the gifts of pork the dispute was then considered to be settled. Great men could also use their powers of intimidation to get people to cooperate, but, of course, this could only work if the other parties were truly intimidated and sometimes they were not.

The status of great man in the Bena Bena was not very precisely defined. It was not always the case that either you were a great man or not in some absolute sense. There were, it is true, certain men that everyone would agree were great men, but there were other men of only slightly lesser stature who might be named only by some as great men. Similarly, when a great man died or was killed another man would emerge as a leader even though he may have been less dominant previously. In cases where no suitable leader was available groups would either attach themselves to the great men of other places or they would disappear. Berndt has described this as it relates to warfare and the scattering of defeated groups in this area of New Guinea: "The weakness here lay in the scattering of power and authority, each village or hamlet, even each lineage, having its leader who remained such until another 'strong' man took his place. There was a more or less constant jockeying for position; and in such a process the system was flexible enough to allow of contrary views and clashes even within the village as well as within the district. The notion of a central authority is in one sense quite contrary to this way of thinking. Although component villages of a district rely to some extent on one another, they rely even more heavily on themselves and on their 'strong' men" (1962:253).[7]

---

7 I realize that in a few Melanesian societies there are "chiefs" rather than merely "great men." However, it appears that even where there are such chiefs they do not wield a great deal of authority and thus, functionally, are not very different from great men. Malinowski says of the Trobriands, for example: ". . . Chieftainship in the Trobriands is the combination of two institutions: first, that of headmanship, or village authority; secondly, that of totemic clanship, that is the division of the community into classes or castes, each with a certain more or less definite rank.

"In every community in the Trobriands, there is one man who wields the greatest authority, though often this does not amount to much" (1922:62). Much the same is true of the people

More importantly, perhaps, with respect to the question of authority, as Bena Bena children were believed to be incapable of reason and virtually unteachable until about seven years of age, such parental authority as existed was seldom invoked over them. And, indeed, even into their teens, male children especially ran wild. They performed no chores, did not help men or women work, and simply ran off with their age mates, playing with bows and arrows and other such pleasurable pursuits. They frequently got into mischief. I know of one case in which a group of boys stoned and killed a man's pig and, although the man was furious, the boys were never punished in any way. Similarly, I observed boys plucking other people's chickens alive in order to get feathers to play with and, again, went unpunished.[8] While it is true to say that a boy's father had authority over him, unlike the case of the Mae Enga (Meggitt 1965) and the Jale (Koch 1974), where paternal punishment could be severe, such authority was rarely invoked in the Bena Bena even when the boy had obviously done something he should not have. Bena Bena fathers were much more prone to defend their children than to punish them no matter what they might have done. But if this situation were allowed to continue indefintely there would, of course, be complete anarchy, a situation which would not bode well for small societies engaged in fights for their very survival. When parents do not discipline their children, and when individual leaders of other kinds also lack the authority to do so, how are succeeding generations socialized into the roles they inevitably must play? Here one sees still another theme of the initiation rites, one which brings into play and features the total and absolute authority of society itself.

In fieldnotes statements I have from Bena Bena informants who were involved in initiations there are recurrent themes.

---

of Waropen (Held 1957) and, indeed, so far as I know for most other such groups who are said to have chiefs.

8 The only two occasions on which I observed children being formally punished both were associated with culture change and had to do with their fear and/or emulation of Europeans.

One of these clearly has to do with the imposition of authority: "You [boys] just ran about and did nothing. You didn't help us. You didn't hear our talk. You didn't bring us water. You didn't help us build houses. You didn't help us in the gardens. You just ran about doing nothing. Now you must hear our talk. Now you must settle down and build houses for your wives and fences for your gardens." These instructions are not given to individual boys by individual men but, rather, are directed at the group of boys by the adult males who are acting as initiators. It is also clear from the actions taken and the tone of voice used that there was a certain amount of hostility on the part of the adult males. And why not? It was true that the boys had in fact done very little constructive work of any kind. This kind of instruction is also found in the Awa case where there is verbal abuse concerning the lack of past helpfulness, instruction about the hard work of gardening, and instruction telling them not to behave as children any longer and do what is commanded of them (Newman and Boyd 1982:250).

I submit that one of the purposes of the rites is to impose authority for the first time upon a group of boys who up until that time had received virtually no discipline of any kind. The authority that is imposed is the absolute and inescapable authority of society itself. And it is imposed in such a dramatic and traumatic way that the message is clear, overwhelming, and never to be forgotten. This would seem to be particularly the case in the Sambia where submitting to the flute sucking is seen as symbolic of submission to authority:

> Though a lad seems to have a choice between orally submitting to and refusing the flute, his sucking behavior reduces him to being a subordinate and, eventually, a fellator, for men clearly state that the act simulates the mechanics of fellation and indicates a boy's willingness to fulfill his erotic role later. Conversely, a novice's refusal signals his defiance of men's authority. We saw how Kokwai responded to this: he entered the ritual scene, followed by several men, all of whom pounded the boys with flutes, making them cry. This "infantile" response was the desired outcome, I think, for the aggressiveness then

> ceased. There, as in secular life, boys who suck the flute are lauded and praised, whereas individuals who reject "it"—authority, status subordination, or fellatio—are scorned, and their resistance tends to induce the men to behave in a hostile manner toward them (Herdt 1982:76).

Serpenti says of Kimam-Papuans, "The attitude of men toward the boy changes radically from the moment he enters the burawa. Before, people had been very indulgent toward children. Now obedience and respect are demanded of initiates, and any infringement of the ritual rules is severely punished, for instance, by beating him with burning sticks . . ." (1984:311). As Poole puts it, "Ritual authority demands respect" (1982:137).

One can see the same power of society mobilized during marriages. It is by no means uncommon for girls to not wish to marry either when or where their legal guardians choose. They complain to their parents, who profess sympathy (and often do, in fact, sympathize with them) but then inevitably add, "You must do what your guardian wishes. That is our way." In this way the entire group stands together against the wishes of the girl and thereby sanctions the marriage. There is nothing the girl can do but comply (except, of course, to attempt to run away *after* she is married, which many do, but not so many succeed).

Because of the nature of Bena Bena childrearing and their beliefs about the nature of children it is perhaps inevitable there should be intergenerational hostility. This expresses itself at times outside of the initiation rites. On many occasions I have observed groups of children playing when, for no apparent reason, an adult male, most usually a younger adult male, suddenly charges into the group, disrupts the game, and disperses the children. They quickly regroup, of course, and then continue what they were doing. I cannot account for this behavior on the part of adults except by assuming they are resentful of the carefree lives of children, a carefree period of life no longer available to adults. It is possible, of course, to argue that this hostility on the part of adult males is attributable to their Oedipal feelings toward their sons. But as I have indicated earlier, I see no basis for Oedipal conflict in the Bena Bena and it is not the fathers who are abusing their sons. I suppose one could argue that the hostility of fathers toward their sons can be displaced onto the sons of others, but that seems to me most unlikely. It appears to me that it is society itself against the undisciplined human raw material that it needs to survive and prosper.

Most basic of all to these rituals is the absolute necessity to create warriors, males willing and able to endure pain and, more importantly perhaps, be able to kill. Indeed, what we now know about New Guinea violence and warfare would lead one to believe that men do not easily or naturally kill and must be well prepared for it. It is true, of course, that some New Guinea societies do not appear to have male initiation rites as such. The Mae Enga, for example, seem to have had a much milder version of initiation associated with the bachelor cults. But with respect to the Mae, at least, one might observe that the combination of their unusually harsh childrearing practices and bachelor cults effectively produced the same results. Mae Enga boys begin staying with their fathers at about age eight. Meggitt says of this:

> More important, of course, is the boy's constant exposure to men's talk and attitudes after he moves into his father's house. Night after night he hears the interminable discussions of political disputes and past battles, the minute dissection of successful and unsuccessful strategies and tactics. In this way he not only learns something of the practice of warfare and the history of his clan's relations with friends and enemies, he also absorbs martial values: he grows up expecting and wanting to be a warrior (1977:62).

When the boy is about fifteen he formally joins the bachelors' association attached to his clan. During this time he learns even more about warfare and begins to participate to gain actual experience in fighting and killing. As the bachelor cults insist on the avoidance of women and also engage in ancestor worship they are in this respect little different from the initiations (see Meggitt, 1977, for the details of all this).

Unlike the Bena Bena and most other Melanesians the Mae Enga are strict and harsh disciplinarians:

> A mild father warns the offending boy once, then punishes him for a repetititon of the misdemeanor, whereas a stern father (and there are many) strikes on the first occasion. The father's punishment can be harsh by Western standards—flogging, tying with pig ropes, smoking the lad for a day over a slow fire, slicing his hand with a knife, or cutting off and cooking his ear lobes and making him eat them so that in the future he will heed his father's commands (1977:195).

Andrew Strathern has written that male initiation ceremonies are absent in the area around Mount Hagen (1970), but Vicedom and Tischner (1943-48(1):242; (2):180-184) claimed that male initiation ceremonies occurred there until the late 1880s (Hays 1985:43; 1986:437). How widespread male initiation rites might have been in New Guinea will never be known due to culture contact in the area before most of the ethnography was done. Most descriptions of the rites make it eminently clear that the initiates were being taught to bear pain stoically and to kill without remorse.

One further aspect of the initiation complex needs to be mentioned. While it has been noted by others that initiation rites are also concerned with education (Barth 1975; Hays and Hays 1982; La Fontaine 1978), most of the literature has ignored this important dimension of them in favor of concentrating on the more exotic and dramatic aspects of the rites, the beatings, purgings, genital mutilations, homosexuality, and the like. Although details are hard to come by, it is certainly the case that a great deal of more mundane information was conveyed to the initiates as well as the sacred lore. In the case of the Bena Bena, initiates were instructed as to precisely who their current and past enemies are and were, they were taught tactics and strategies for fighting, including such things as proper house construction (which would allow people to escape from their houses). They were taught the names of the 50 or so different types of arrows, how best to make them, and so forth. They were instructed in husbandly duties beyond the specific matters of sex. They were told how to treat guests and affines. They were instructed in their history and in the men's secrets having to do with the flutes, the *nama* (the giant bird that was said to make the sound of the flutes), the bull-roarer, and other such things. In addition they were taught love magic to make them attractive to women, magic to protect themselves from women, magic to protect themselves from their enemies, and so on. They also learned their cultural beliefs about the nature of conception and the differences between men and women.

If we see the various Bena Bena initiation ceremonies as a sequence beginning when boys are about five or six years of age and have their ears pierced and ending only after they are married and have children, which seems to have been the case, it is clear that their instruction took place over a period of many years. Even though Bena youths were apparently actually secluded for shorter periods of time than others, their instruction obviously continued between the initiation ceremonies while they were living with the men in the men's house. Even when the boys were not being subjected to the actual physical elements of initiation they were still being instructed in these other matters, instructions that were periodically reinforced through the traumatic rites.

The educational aspects of the initiation complex should not be underestimated. There was a great deal to learn:

> Religious, initiatory, and economic activities were complementary to fighting, and settlement patterns and construction organized in relation to defense and attack. Socialization included not simply training boys in the techniques or arts of warfare, but also their persistent indoctrination in the appropriate beliefs and assumptions. War-magic, or sorcery, was a widespread feature of this complex. The material weapons involved in fighting—bow and arrows, shields and clubs—took much time and energy to prepare; in the Eastern Highlands, for instance, arrow types were individually named, and in fact arrows were far more decorative and more carefully made than the sacred flutes. Songs and myths relating to war are a topic in themselves (Berndt 1964:185).

Newman and Boyd have given perhaps the most detailed account of the educational aspects of initiation. In the Awa case it is clear that although the initiation deals with physiological maturity, it also deals importantly with the assumption of increasingly adult social responsibilities (1982:245). For example, the first of the Awa rites, the "sugarcane rite," emphasizes how hard it is to grow sugarcane and instructs the boys that it is an adult responsibility they must now accept (1982:248). Then they are scraped raw on the thighs by two men pulling a rough vine back and forth between their legs. This is to instruct them not to be afraid of climbing trees when looking for marsupials or when cutting branches of trees for use in their gardens (1982:250). The boys are later "shown the garden." Uncooked yams, taro, sweet potatoes, bananas, and the like are displayed in a large pile in the men's house. They are told they can no longer play about the gardens in a childish manner. At this time they are dressed in an entirely new manner and told they must conduct themselves in a quiet, dignified manner rather than running about like children (1982:250).

Newman and Boyd say of this first stage of initiation: "This first phase in the initiation sequence most obviously concerns effecting a separation of the initiates from the pursuits and relationships of childhood and directing their attention to the importance of achieving the physical growth, the strength, and the social commitment toward men deemed necessary in adult life. These matters are mostly a background in the consciousness of the boys, who experience the ritual primarily as frightening and painful and who are full of uncertainty about what may happen to them. Nevertheless, the ritual does introduce them in dramatic fashion to fundamental ideas. In the period between their induction and the next major ritual, they eat the solid garden foods that build firm bodies, draw away from the attachments of childhood, and begin participating in the work activities of adult males if only in small ways. The ritual also sets a pattern for later rituals in the sequence, and as the initiates pass through the whole process, the adult meaning of many of the elements in this rite are brought more fully into their awareness" (1982:251-52).

The next ritual in the Awa initiation sequence, which involves a beating or beatings, likewise emphasizes social responsibility:

> This beating, unlike the beating with nettles administered in the preceding ritual, is not connected with inducing physical growth, but is instead linked to ideas of social responsibility within the patriclan. The emotional atmosphere in the men's house is highly charged at this point as individual kinsmen of the initiates (frequently elder brothers) sporadically begin recounting misdeeds that a particular boy has committed in the past, such as stealing or causing a fight. These harangues rise in crescendos of anger as the older men push to the center of the house and thrash the youths in retaliation for their transgressions. It is not only transgressors who are beaten, however, for blows are also administered in the name of men killed in warfare or as retribution for wounds inflicted on the living while they protected the initiates when the latter were too small to aid the group in its own defense. Thus, all initiates are beaten, whether they have been transgressors or not. In this manner they are forcefully instructed regarding both their obligation to act responsibly toward clan members in the future and their duty to become strong enough to help defend the group against attack from outside (1982:252-53).

Awa initiation rites, like those of other Eastern Highlanders, are concerned with sexual behavior, procreation, and protection from pollution. However, instruction in these matters does not take place until the fourth and fifth stages of initiation, as the earlier stages concentrate on physical growth and adult social obligations (1982:283).

While the sequences may not be identical everywhere in New Guinea, it is likely the case that the rites served much the same educational purposes everywhere. Hays and Hays, for example, mention that "Both of these transitions are marked by major ceremonies, after which both sexes begin periods of extensive instruction and preparation for adult roles" (1982:208), but they do not elaborate on this except for discussions of procreation, sex, gender, and pollution. The emphasis on adult responsibility is found among the Baruya as well:

> At the moment when, standing motionless and silent . . . the master of this ceremony delivers a long speech to remind them that henceforward they are men, that soon their elders will be finding wives for them, but the task will be a difficult one if the fathers of marriageable daughters learn that so and so is lazy or a thief. He reminds them that, once married, they will have to clear the forest and lay out gardens to feed their family, that they will be expected to fulfill all their responsibilities toward their wives, children, to all their consanguine relatives or affines. Above all, they must henceforward be prepared to fight to the death to defend the Baruya and their territory (Godelier 1986:35).

More precisely it is pointed out that "Every Baruya is a warrior, hunter, and horticulturalist. The initiations and the community life that the Baruya impose on boys for a period of over ten years are precisely designed to turn each of them into a man competent in all three areas" (1986:97).

As Meggitt observed, for the Kuma the rites are primarily didactic: "Moreover, although in one respect such initiation symbolizes the separation of the lads from the mothers, its purpose is primarily didactic—the inculcation of clan values. 'Lecturers instruct the novices to cooperate in work with clansmen; to marry and have sons to continue their line; to be strong and defeat the clan's enemies, avenge the death of a clansman, and prevent the clan from being destroyed. In short, they must do as their fathers did'" (1964:220). Enga fathers educate their sons in much the same ways without the formal initiation rites (Meggitt 1977).

Lawrence describes the educational and leadership aspects of Garia initiation rites as follows:

> In Garia eyes, however, the overriding importance of initiation is religious rather than social: the introduction of youths to the realm of superhuman beings so that they have the opportunity to acquire "true" knowledge, not the mere secular skills they have previously gleaned but the lore of ghosts and deities. Youths are placed under the protection of their immediate forebears, and are progressively taught the myths and ritual that will grant them beneficial relationships with particular deities within their

> political regions. . . . At first, a boy's instruction is only general and, should he show no aptitude or ambition, it will never be more. Yet should he aspire to leadership, it becomes more intensive, especially after he has participated fully in the Abaiwala ceremoney. Whereas unmotivated youths now drop out, he will undergo, outside formal intitiation, special periods of serious religious tuition. . . . Normally, provided he has the requisite knowledge, a father will be his sons' first teacher: he will instruct them in the myths for the creation of the physical environment and human beings, but more particularly in myths and ritual for the two initiation ceremonies, their bush god(s), and deities for food plants, livestock, artefacts and dances. But a youth may not be restricted to only one teacher or set of ritual formulae. He may turn to older agnates, who may have greater learning than his father (1984:212-13).

Van Baal, writing of the Marind-anim, says that "The *mayo*-initiation provided an almost complete re-training. From our sources we gather that only few aspects of life were left out, and from the paucity of these sources we may conclude that the extent of the education given is more comprehensive than appears from our enumeration of the successive episodes" (1966:544).

It seems clear enough that male initiation rites in the New Guinea Highlands do in fact have a great deal to do with the control of sexuality and procreation, leadership and authority, and, more broadly, enculturation in general, including enculturation for warriorhood. As Herdt has said: "Initiation makes all men warriors" (1981:52). But the rites have significance far beyond any of this as in their entirety they organize and define the social order itself. As Whitehead has put it: ". . . We will find in ritual as well the articulation of those principles in terms of which solidarity and alliance are culturally understood, principles such as . . . manhood and clanhood. This is the case not just because ritual reflects the social order but because, in most areas of New Guinea, ritual quite literally composes the social order" (1986:86).

7
Conclusions

It is not at all surprising that there is a considerable amount of variation involved in the literature of New Guinea having to do with the interpretation of initiation rites, procreation, blood, semen, and other things. New Guinea is a vast island with a long history of human settlement and, by now, a fairly long history of ethnographic research. As Barth has shown, there is variation from place to place in New Guinea cosmologies simply as a result of the fact that the ritual knowledge is held in the memories of only a few individuals who are asked to employ it only infrequently. Because of this and the nature of small groups relatively isolated from each other it is not surprising that this should be so (Barth 1987). Feil has shown that in the Highlands case there have been different evolutionary histories from east to west (1987).

That there is considerable variation is indisputable; in some areas there are initiation rites which are absent in others, homosexuality exists in one society and a short distance away a similar group knows nothing of it, some are matrilineal and others patrilineal, most groups seem to believe semen creates bone but in a few others people say it is blood that does so, and so on. But there is also a question as to how much of this variation might be the result simply of the fact that ethnographic work was carried out at different periods of time and by anthropologists of different theoretical persuasions and training, different political views, different genders, and even different sexual preferences. There are also problems of more or less missionary activity, language, and translation.

There is a further problem in that most of the anthropological observations in New Guinea were made after changes had occurred so aboriginal cultures were not as they originally were. Thus, as in the case of the Hageners, we cannot know for certain in all cases whether initiation rites might have occurred or not, nor can we know how drastically local exegeses might have been affected by contact. Furthermore, anthropologists do not often report the absence of traits so that, for example, if no mention is made of beliefs about bone marrow or bloodletting, that does not mean they might not have existed. In spite of all these problems, however, there is remarkable agreement on the widespread presence of many important features of these cultures: clan exogamy, violence and warfare, male superiority, avoidance of menstrual blood, initiation and/or puberty rites or something resembling them, the use of semen in such rites, bloodletting, genital "operations," sacred flutes, a concern with the regulation of sexuality, separation of the sexes, and amorphous ancestral cults.

There is, of course, variation even with respect to these traits. It is difficult to determine in most cases how much of it is real. For example, how does one determine just how polluting something is believed to be? If men sleep in the same house with their wives and children does that imply that women there are less polluting than elsewhere? How do you determine how much contact really exists between fathers and their children? And what about the quality of that contact? How do you know just how rampant warfare actually was and how can you readily compare one New Guinea society with another on these dimensions? How do you determine just how "inferior" women are believed to be? How do you really determine whether or not sons "hate" their fathers and "love" their mothers? While we make these claims and attempt such comparisons, I submit they may well be erroneous or at best perhaps only partial truths. We cannot merely accept every ethnographic claim as valid without question. With this in mind what can we make of what we do know?

Women, in this scheme of things, are often considered not only hypersexual but also potentially untrustworthy, unpredictable, transitory, and dispensable; here today, gone tomorrow. In the majority of New Guinea cultures not only were women strangers to their husbands and their people, as wives residing in their husbands' clans they were strangers even to each other. Unlike male agnates, women had divided loyalties and could be torn between the demands of husbands and brothers, husbands' and fathers' clans.[1] Furthermore, where divorce was so common and sorcery or witchcraft so suspect, women could be seen as potentially even more dangerous and unreliable. Even the female contribution to life was believed to be impermanent. Blood and flesh disappear. The only things that remained and had any genuine continuity were male: male solidarity and bone. But, at the same time, women were always there, living in the villages but not really of them, excluded from male initiation rites but still part of them, disenfranchised but still influential, expendable but absolutely necessary, feared but still desired, and even loved. So what were people to do?

What people did, it appears, motivated by necessity and bound by beliefs perhaps only partially understood but handed down over countless generations, was band together in the interests of human and group fertility and continuity.

---

[1] There are, of course, cases where village endogamy is common and other cases where women do not necessarily come as brides from distant places. How much difference this may make with respect to various attitudes and behaviors is largely unknown. Newman, for example, comparing Gururumba and Awa, suggests that the presence of beliefs about female witches in the former may be related to the fact that women are strangers to their husband's groups whereas in Awa, because they marry nearby, women are not designated as witches. Awa women also appear to have somewhat more power to collectively defend themselves than do Gururumba women but other than that there seem to be few if any significant differences in beliefs and practices having to do with women, initiates, and so forth. (1981:115).

But, as fertility and continuity were perceived primarily as male, in doing so they could not be unaware of the existence of "woman." The contributions of the female of the species to procreation and, indeed, to the general well-being of others, could hardly be denied. There are, as we have seen, different attempts to accomodate the contributions of women, most usually by claiming that women merely carry the child that men have created. Beyond this, however, it appears that the major contribution woman made, apart from her unique capacity to bear children, however unconscious, subconscious, symbolic, or otherwise buried in the cultural tradition it may have been, was to acknowledge the necessity for community and thus continuity. One might argue that in the interests of social order and safety woman surrendered her power to men.[2] Errington makes a statement very much to this effect:

> I suggest that the *kavei* [a ceremony involving shell money] is a statement to women that they are still, as they were at one time, capable of upholding rather than subverting order. . . . The "women of the *tubuan*" [female ritual figure] have committed themselves during the kavei to upholding social order. As "mothers," they have accepted the constraints of *divara* [shell money] and moiety in bride price and marriage; as "mothers," their sexuality is focused on reproduction, which strengthens rather than divides society; as "mothers," they accept the male perspective by supporting their sons in becoming adepts; as supporters of their sons they are supporting with divara the principle that social order is based on divara. . . .
>
> The kavei is in part, I suggest, an effort to make women controllable: to induce them, by accepting divara, to allow themselves to be ordered by it. By thus accepting divara as the standard of order they would support social order as they once did when they controlled the tubuan and acted as adepts . . . (1974:119-20).

I suggest that men in other New Guinea cultural groups admitted the same thing symbolically by acknowledging that

---

2 For an account of how women can ruin men if they wish see Errington and Gewertz: ". . . Mead is correct when she suggests that Chambri men recognize that their security depends upon women: the security, however, stems less from the emotional support women may provide than for their women remaining politically disengaged" (1987:80).

originally the flutes and their attendant power were in the hands of women. Thus, even if women were disenfranchised at the moment, it had not always been so and was for just cause.[3] I do not believe it is true that ". . . in central Wahgi societies . . . the value of women is recognized and accurately assessed for the first time" (Feil 1987:220).[4] It is interesting to note that although the myths indicate that the flutes were originally in the hands of women and subsequently stolen or otherwise acquired by men, there is rarely any explanation offered for why this happened.

As it appears to be the case that motives are not always offered in either New Guinea folktales or myths (Newman 1990), perhaps this is understandable. That is, the motives or reasons involved are apparently obvious to the listeners and need not be specified. If that be so, in the case of the flute myths, it would seem obvious that men would of course take from women anything of importance which they did not otherwise possess. What is more interesting, perhaps, is that it is never very seriously suggested that women might attempt to get the flutes back.[5] This might well be interpreted as their acquiescence to the status quo. Hays and Hays have said it well:

> Why do Ndumba women thus actively cooperate in the performance of ceremonies whose central meanings consign them to subservient positions in society and whose main theme appears to be misogynistic? If the 'ummanra and kwaasi ceremonies have at their core the assertion of men's power, they also imply women's acceptance of that social imbalance.

3 Andrew Strathern, writing of a Female Spirit Cult, makes the following interpretation: "My explanation of the spirit's paradoxical nature is thus that men, in their image of her, project a notion of an unthreatening female, who can, in fact, protect them against the threat represented by their true wives. She is beautiful, as a young bride can be, but benign too, for her genitals are forever closed. She does not bear children, but she guarantees fertility. In seeing her as female at all, the men, I suggest, are also covertly admitting the importance of their wives as bearers of fertility" (1970:583).

4 I do not know what is meant by "accurately" here but certainly the value of women is "recognized" in the Eastern Highlands and elsewhere if not in precisely the same ways.

5 For an excellent review of flute myths and associated behaviors see Hays 1988.

> . . . Far from being simply a misogynistic male belief, the postulation of fundamental male-female differences that are dangerous to men and thus problematic for society may be seen as a contention shared by men and women alike. The need to exert control over women's powers is acknowledged by both sexes; the institutional mechanisms for doing so are firmly grounded. To possess such awesome forces is a heavy responsibility and, perhaps, one that carries its own satisfactions. When a Ndumba woman prepares her son for initiation or instructs her daughter in the new powers of her body, "it would seem that, as a conscious human and member of culture, she has followed out the logic of culture's arguments and has reached culture's conclusions along with the men" (Ortner 1974:76) (1982:237).[6]

Weston La Barre has informed us, in his fascinating work, *Muelos,* of a stone-age superstition about sexuality that has survived from the Paleolithic to the present. I suggest this may well be relevant here. It is a belief in the power of semen and a type of "bone cult" virtually as old as mankind. It is an explanation for life and consciousness:

> Animistic belief in a separable soul, besides explaining life and death, serves also to explain the mysterious persistent *patterning* in animals, since no matter how many individual animals are killed by hunters, and their flesh eaten by the people, the animal species remains abundant, in a kind of immortal *logos*-pattern that remains unchanged—a mysterious principle, evidently male, inherent in bones, the fundamental framework for life. For it can easily be observed that only through the intervention of a male principle is reproduction possible, the supposed stamping of pattern upon formless materia-substance. The growth of a child in a woman's body is no mystery. The increment comes from the food the mother eats, quite as later growth comes from the milk she gives her child. The mystery lies in the inception of life: consciousness, life, warmth appear to be a male gift, and surely from his semen (1984:2).

In this archaic belief system bones are the framework of life but more specifically it is the semenlike marrow (*muelos*) in the bones that is believed to be the source of semen. "The skull, as the bone enclosing the most plentiful *muelos*-marrow

---

6 I do not believe this has to refer exclusively to "women's powers" but, rather, to reproductive power and fertility in general.

in the body (the brain), is therefore the major repository of the generative life-stuff or semen" (1984:3).

In its basic fundamentals there need be no denigration of females as such in this ancient belief system. It asserts simply (and however controversial it may be) that the power of creation and the continuity of the human species is the result of male attributes. The place for woman in this scheme is enigmatic and open to a wide variety of explanations and interpretations thus posing some of the "conundrums in our understanding both of the New Guinea materials and of 'male dominance' generally" (Whitehead 1986a:273). This is precisely why Marilyn Strathern can point to the ethnocentricity of the proposition "Women make babies" (1988:311). In New Guinea it appears that it is men who make babies, women merely carry them. Marilyn Strathern asks ". . . Yet if the houses are decorated with figures whose appendages can be read as both breasts and phalluses, then what is 'male' and what is 'female' in the first place? Is the phallus a male breast? Is it to emphasize its maleness or femaleness that the breast is imagined as a female phallus?" (1988:126). The answer, I think, is that it doesn't matter, they are all symbols of fertility, and fertility is understood to be fundamentally male. As in Sambia, "the woman's body is thus regarded as a transformer of male substance" (M. Strathern 1988:217). Similarly, among the Bimin-Kuskusmin: ". . . male agnates of a dead woman eat fragments of her bone marrow to re-absorb the fertile fluids that they have procreatively transmitted to her at conception. Through subsequent ritual acts and the consumption of *finiik*-bearing male foods, they will transform her bone marrow and fertile fluids into semen in their own bodies" (Poole 1984:209).

As woman exists, both males and females have had to confront this basic and somewhat paradoxical fact. As it is for the Bedamini, I suggest, so it is for the rest of Papua New Guinea: "The men, in their own eyes, ultimately possess the power, and the responsibility, of the reproduction of mankind and the cosmos, but they cannot, socially or ideologically, escape their dependence on women" (Sorum 1982:61). Given the basic beliefs about male fertility the existence of woman creates what Jorgensen has termed a patrilineal puzzle: ". . . Society as a symbolically masculine construction rests upon the premise that women's procreative capacities are at once foundational and problematic, a state of affairs that makes the ideological life of these societies tricky" (1983:4). I suggest it is, however, because *male procreative powers are foundational* that the position of women becomes so problematical. Given this situation it is not surprising to find considerable variation in the way woman's contribution is explained. That is, as merely transformational, an incubator, a temporary home, the contributor of blood, or, in rare circumstances, bone. Matrilineality, I suggest, makes no real difference here other than perhaps somewhat more publicly enhancing the status of women. The basic transactions in matrilineal societies, as in patrilineal ones, are not between women and men but between mother's brothers and sister's sons. Even in the Trobriands it is not the daughters who "suck their father's bones" (again, see Glass 1996).

Male dominance, it must be pointed out, is a necessity in this belief system. If fertility is male, and if the continuity of life and perhaps nature itself is dependent upon the production and transmission of this vital male principle, all else, including women, must be made to serve this sacred purpose. The "apparently inexplicable question of motive [which] dogs the question of male domination" (M. Strathern 1988:93), simply disappears as does "the unanswerable question [of Levi-Strauss and others], how do men obtain this right?" (Whitehead 1986:287).

By concentrating primarily on the initiation rites alone, or only on certain selected topics such as power, gender, homosexuality, male-female relations, and so on, we have erred in our studies of male initiation rites by failing to see them in this larger context. Annette Weiner is quite right on this point:

> Reproduction must be understood as more than biological processes and more than "social reproduction" in a Marxist context. For reproduction includes more than giving birth, and more than the reproduction of social relations. Reproduction pertains to the particular form in which individuals are tied to each other and the way these ties are expressed through the exchange of substances, materials, and knowledge. The work and production necessary to express these ties ultimately represent the labour necessary to document, and thus validate, the regeneration of some form or rebirth following death (1982:64).

This is not, then, a question of males, bloated by self-importance, merely joining together to imitate childbirth and dominate women, nor is it simply a conspiracy of males intent on creating a world without women. It is certainly not, in Wagner's flippant view, simply ". . . a kind of collective effort by the second best sex to corner its meat supply . . ."(1983:77). Seen in their broader context the rites speak directly to the same fundamental cosmological and existential problems as all other religions.[7] They appear to be a classic example of an ancestral bone cult based upon beliefs so archaic as to be buried deep within the cultural unconscious. And it is here the great paradox lies: culture makes demands the heart cannot accept. While a world of males is prescribed by the belief system, the existence, nature, necessity, and desirability of "woman" simply could not be denied.

It is an interesting fact of New Guinea anthropology that when writing specifically on religion the emphasis is primarily on supernatural beings and the initiations are hardly mentioned (Lawrence and Meggitt 1965; Herdt and Stephen 1989), whereas those studying the initiations barely mention super-

[7] One explanation for this may have to do with the fact that much of the anthropological work in Melanesia has been carried out relatively recently during a period in which anthropologists have tended to focus much more on specific issues rather than larger ethnographic works. This can be seen if one compares recent anthropological work to that of earlier Melanesian ethnographers. On the part of some it may have had to do with ethnocentrism: ". . . However, except for certain higher religions and for persons capable of very abstract conceptual ways of thinking, the difference between right or wrong and good or evil may be a matter of cultural mores" (Lidz and Lidz 1989:39).

natural beings other than ancestors.[8] Barth's study of Baktaman ritual and knowledge is somewhat of an exception. He makes what I believe is the crucial point: "I should emphasize the character of Baktaman religion as a communal cult run by men, not a male cult; to the best of my knowledge there is no counterbalancing female cult, and the few ritual activities of women are mostly derivative from, or minor elements in, the male-run cult activities" (1975:24). J. Weiner makes a similar observation: "Thus, although the rituals of the Usi resemble at many points an initiation programme for adolescent boys, this is not its intent or primary goal in Foi male thinking. It is more a competitive appropriation of ghostly power by men, deployed for both collective and individual benefit" (1987:275).

This suggests what appears to be a common pattern in which cultural constraints fashioned in antiquity and situationally promoted over a long period of time conflicted with basic biological urges. The result of this was a powerful ambivalence in the relationships of women to men which, in turn, created a number of cultural paradoxes. For example, in such a belief system the very fact that women desire and/or seek sexual gratification at all is evidence of their wanton character. If a woman attempted to get her husband or lover to prolong the sex act for her enjoyment this was further confirmation of her unbridled sexuality. And men, culturally programmed to think of women and sex as dangerous and polluting, must have found their own biologically based desires in conflict with their culturally prescribed beliefs (and perhaps their ability to perform?). The drive for sex, and thus for female companionship and yes, I would say family as well, was artifically

---

[8] It is also interesting that works on Melanesian religions tend not to feature what might be seen as the more "exotic" aspects of them such as the smearing of semen, eating of brain, bloodletting, group intercourse, sucking the bones of the dead, and so forth. Could it be the case that dealing with these matters might have rendered New Guinea religions like ". . . all primitive religions . . . grotesque and . . . unintelligible" as Morgan claimed so long ago? (1877:5).

thwarted by a series of beliefs which, however irrational or nonrational, "made sense" in the larger context of their lives.

In this system of belief it was bone, created by semen, that was the only substance of permanence and thus the foundation for the continuity of generations. But it became the obligation of both men *and* women to insure that continuity, and insofar as semen was male, it was primarily males who were involved. Thus the rites were not "merely a charade" but, rather, an obligation of men that was also recognized by women who "went along with it," not out of coercion or fear, but because of the force of culture itself. They understood that the rites were for them as well as for males. Watson suggests this for the Tairora: "We are speaking of a culture in which the membership and participation of males is emphasized, in which their masculinity is an undeniable preoccupation of the community at large—indeed, one of its major resources—and one where the community itself is in some sense patrilineally organized" (1983:255).

In order to believe interpretations of New Guinea initiation rites based upon concepts like Oedipal conflict, womb envy, or even concepts like gender anxiety, one must believe that the people in question do not really believe in their own beliefs. The Oedipal hypothesis implies that the local beliefs about the maturation of youths, the nature of women, the facts of procreation, and so forth, are not a sufficient explanation for the performance of the rites. The belief in womb envy implies that men do not really believe in their own superiority, fertility, and power. The belief in gender-identity confusion implies that they do not believe in their beliefs about the differences between boys and girls and in the different treatment they are accorded virtually from birth.

The argument from pre-Oedipal experience to faulty gender identification to homosexuality implies that the people involved do not believe in their beliefs about male maturation. To argue that men envy wombs or giving birth implies that they do not really believe that menstruation and childbirth are polluting. Let me repeat the example from Meigs:

> It should be emphasized that *kupa* [male pregnancy] is a feared and an abhorred condition. Yet one cannot resist suggesting that it is also desired. All the facts deny the premise that males can become pregnant. I submit that the reason males believe they can become pregnant, and belief in the fake fetuses provided by the curers, is that they have strong psychological reasons to do so. They have a will to believe that they are fertile (1984:55).

As we have seen, however, in this belief system it is males who are fertile and who must insure the fertility of females. Related here is the belief of Bena Bena and probably most other New Guineans that males cannot be sterile. That is, if a man has no children it is never because of some fault of his but, rather, that his wife or wives are somehow preventing him from doing so.

Still another problem with the existing interpretations has to do with the imposition of theory on data. Stoller and Herdt, for example, attempt to explain Sambia homosexuality the way they explain it in the United States; that is, ineffective and absent fathers. But Sambia, as Herdt and Stoller are well aware, are not homosexuals in the same way those seeking help through Western psychiatry are. One might well argue that Sambia homosexuality is explained simply through their belief system—they do it because they believe they have to do it if they are to properly mature.[9] Similarly, Lidz and Lidz (1989) attempt to apply a hypothesis to New Guinea derived from the pathological behavior of a few Western European children observed by Bettelheim (1954). But why, if Papua New Guineans do believe what they claim to believe about men and women, procreation, and so forth, would men have any reason to envy females? Given the beliefs in the overwhelming superiority of men, how could they have developed

---

9 It is interesting that Herdt and Stoller, although they employ the Oedipal hypothesis, tend to emphasize the pre-Oedipal phase. I assume this has to do with the fact that a full-blown Oedipal complex, resolved, would be fundamentally inconsistent with the notion of faulty gender identification.

faulty gender identity? It is possible to argue, of course, that this was a case of reaction formation because men unconsciously envied females. But then where was the source of their unconscious beliefs? If one believes that the content of the unconscious is the result of culturally repressed materials, where did such materials exist in the culture? If my interpretation here is correct it appears that several generations of anthropologists in New Guinea may have repeatedly made the most basic of ethnocentric errors. Namely, assuming that it must be believed that it is females who hold the key to human reproduction because they give birth. But there are few, if any, earth mothers or madonnas in Melanesian religions. Fertility as a male principle has been virtually ignored; but see Collier and Rosaldo (1981) and Lutkehaus (1995).

I see no reason to assume that Bena Bena males and other Highlanders were not doing more or less exactly what they professed to be doing; that is, celebrating and reaffirming the essentially male powers that both created and sustained human life as well as worshipping and emulating the procreative powers of nature in general.[10] There are many statements indicating this in the literature. For example: "Although it is with their *min* (their mortal life stuff) that men invest the *rumbim*, it may be that the association of *min* with agnatic corporations imbues the commingled *min* which infuses the *rumbim* with, if not immortality, a perdurance beyond that of individual lives. By clasping *rumbim*, a man participates in a life whose span is greater than his own" (Buchbinder and Rappaport 1976:28). Where else but in New Guinea could a leader

[10]Perhaps regeneration is a better word than procreation. Gell, for example, says: ". . . As a fertility ritual *ida* does not promote fertility so much as 'normalize' it, that is to say *ida* is an acting out of the processes of natural and social regeneration in such a way as to place those processes in a framework of symbolic categories. It is an act of participation in these processes; a dramatic performance which runs in parallel to the performances mounted by nature herself" (1975:223). There is perhaps no better account of the importance of males to fertility and regeneration and the use of phallic rituals to that end than Gell's marvelously detailed analysis of the "*ida*" ritual in *Metamorphosis of the Cassowaries* (1975).

stand forth and proclaim, "I have eaten of my father's cock," and have it greeted with "cheers and whooping" (Sorum 1982:53).

Newman and Boyd postulate no Oedipal problems or faulty gender identity but view Awa initiation rites ". . . as a ritual setting in which young men are taught the nature of cosmic forces influencing growth and procreation and the techniques used by men to manipulate and control these processes. The forces that dominate the processes of physical growth, the maintenance of physical well-being, and the achievement of reproductive success are manipulated by the exertion of control over the growth-inducing, generative processes and bodily substances associated with the procreative powers of *both men and women*" (1982:242). The serial intercourse a new bride must endure with her husband's senior patrikin is done to "protect the well-being of their younger male kin and *promote the successful reproduction of their group*. . . . Inflicting pain on the genitalia of young women, as on those of young men, is said to strengthen reproductive organs and stimulate the production of bodily substances associated with procreation" (1982:282).[11]

Gillison, too, describes the overwhelming male emphasis of the rites:

> The debasement of Gimi women cannot be attributed to their symbolic association with the surrounding rainforest because that realm is regarded as a male refuge from women and from ordinary life within the settlement. The Gimi wilderness is an exalted domain where the male spirit, incarnate in birds and marsupials, acts out its secret desires away from the inhibiting presence of women. Gimi men's mundane existence is degraded and their mortal potential is unfulfilled because of the inescapable nearness of women inside the hamlet and of the powerful contamination which female sexuality exudes . . . men's ambition, as expressed in their rituals, is to identify with the non-human world and to be revitalized by its limitless, masculine powers (1980:143-44).

While it is true that the male rituals insure that power re-

[11]Emphases are mine.

mains in the hands of men, as I and others have argued in the past, that power is not simply the power to command women but is, in addition and in fact, the power to insure the fertility and well-being of both males and females as well as nature itself. Hays has said it very well:

> I have argued that the flutes may be interpreted as representing powers of fertility and growth, and that in one set of objects Highlands men have ingeniously combined phallic, bird, and wind symbolism of a kind used all over the world for this purpose. Postulating that women were the original possessors of such instruments may be no more than a metaphoric acknowledgement of women's natural procreative capacities (1988:114).[12]

Sorum has summed it up more simply: ". . . The men, in their own eyes, ultimately possess the power, and the responsibility, of the reproduction of mankind and the cosmos, but they cannot, socially or ideologically, escape their dependence on women" (1982:61). Lewis has said of the Gnau: "The rites of puberty are not solely secular but draw on powers associated with great spirits and unnamed spirits; they are addressed not only to this world of the living but also to the dead. And the men have responsibility for their proper performance, a responsibility and capacity to fulfil these duties restricted to them, and given value by secrecy" (1980:185). It is perhaps because men are in a different (and higher?) state of being (Herdt:1990a) that they are therefore obligated all the more to insure the health, fertility, well-being, and continuity of their particular groups.

But of course, as Robbins hinted about Auyana men, there *is* one way in which men might be said to envy woman. It does not involve wanting to *be* a woman, nor does it involve wishing to menstruate or bear children. It involves the desire to escape the difficult, demanding, and treacherous world of males necessitated by the continuing violence, the desire to be "garden men" (Robbins 1982:190). Is it at all surprising that

[12] I confess it is a mystery to me why females' procreative capacities are any more "natural" than those of males.

little boys cry for their mothers and later, as men, think back fondly of the time they were relatively free of fear and the awesome duties and responsibilities of warfare? Although Bena Bena men occasionally reminisced about their war experiences, without exception they did not want to return to the precontact situation, "the good old days," if you will. The implications of this are profound, for it suggests that although humans are by nature aggressive, as indeed they must be to survive in the world, they are not, by nature, killers of each other. As can be seen by the violence of the rites involved, New Guineans had to work very hard to make their boys not only into men, but into warriors. At bottom, in addition to whatever else was involved, there can be no doubt that the rites were specifically intended, among other things, for this purpose.

There is considerable evidence that this was so. Barth writes, for example:

> . . . There are strong suggestions in the way informants recount wars that there is at the time of battle a considerable atmosphere of fierceness, anger and excitement; but fear seems the more prevalent emotion associated with violence. This attitude toward warfare is also very clearly revealed by the response to the mere declaration of pacification on first contact; no aggressive acts between communities have subsequently taken place. Even when telling about successful raids informants are more prone to praise the present peace than express nostalgia for the pre-contact insecurity, in contrast to their positive attitude to other pre-contact features, such as health and taro size (1975:153).

Robbins comments similarly for Auyana:

> The attitude of men toward fighting varied. I do not know how much of what was said to me would have been said before the arrival of the government. I doubt that I would have been told then, as I was a few times, that fighting was *totally* bad and resulted in nothing but killing and more killing. I do not, however, think it was mere rhetoric when I was told life was better since the government had come because a man could now eat without looking over his shoulder and could leave his house in the morning to urinate without fear of being shot. All men admitted that they were afraid when they fought. In fact, they usually looked at me as though I were a mental defective

> for even asking. Men admitted having nightmares in which they became totally isolated from others in their group during a fight and could see no way back (1982:189).

Even among the Jale: "While in their songs and boastful speeches the Jale praise their bellicose stance and military feats and extol the pleasures of eating enemies and their pigs, in a more reflective mood several of their best warriors have told me that fighting is a 'bad thing'" (Koch, in Knauft 1990:288). Read, in commenting on the changes that occurred for the Gahuku-Gama, suggests that men as well as women were liberated by pacification:

> The cultural "forcing" of human material to fit approved gender identities requires controls and the limiting of expression on both sexes alike; and with Gahuku these were applied in many ways with equal harshness. If women's choices were limited, so were those of men; and, indeed, there was a greater problem in producing the proper gender identity from male material, necessitating undeniably violent and traumatic rites and, thereafter, extreme forms of self-discipline to maintain it. It is quite apparent that many men did not willingly submit to the straightjacket of Gahuku masculinity, any more than numbers of males in our own culture have been or are completely comfortable in the particular jacket they are required to wear (1982:77).[13]

But if it is true that New Guineans truly held these beliefs which were so central to their lives and, indeed, constituted what I have labeled their "religious system,"[14] why did they give them up so easily after contact with Europeans? There are three reasons for this: (1) When warfare and raiding were outlawed the most fundamental necessity for the rites disappeared and men's basic biological desires for women and children which had been held in check, as well as their desire

[13]Whitehead makes an interesting comment which is relevant here: ". . . These women and children, along with their menfolk, lie under shared peril from the weapons of the enemy outsider, against whom the men constitute themselves as the primary protection. Men die in this valiant duty; how then can one accuse them of selfish interests" (1986a:279).

[14]Obviously New Guineans do not divide their beliefs and behaviors up into categories like "religion," "education," "economics," and so forth. My point in doing this here is to emphasize that the whole process of birth and life and death is the basic context in which all of these various elements combine.

to escape the culturally constituted male role, were allowed to be expressed more freely. (2) The functions the rites performed having to do with the control of sexuality, leadership, and authority, and education in general were *all* taken over more or less simultaneously by the new system that was introduced. (3) The most basic beliefs about the importance and superiority of males were in most respects still congruent with those of the new and dominant culture. It might be pointed out that in spite of the fact that after contact women were technically given more legal protection they were often treated just as disrespectfully by some European prospectors, planters, and patrol officers as they might have been aboriginally. Administrative control by no means brought about equal rights for females.

Some will no doubt think I have grossly overgeneralized in these comments on the ethnography of New Guinea. Perhaps I have. Certainly it is the case that not all New Guinea cultures have male initiation rites. But in attempting to understand the foundations upon which they seem to be based it appears they, just as the homosexuality that sometimes accompanies them, are merely one element in a much larger and much more widely shared system of belief which in its fundamentals can be seen as religious. The beliefs about semen, bone, blood, and the fundamental superiority of males were quite likely ubiquitous throughout all of New Guinea, a type of "Ur culture," if you will, from which variations began to appear over time.[15]

It is not surprising that local exegeses vary somewhat in their beliefs about these things, nor is it surprising that leadership varies somewhat from place to place, or that exchanges are on a grander scale in some areas. As Feil has shown, for example, agricultural practices evolved at different rates in

[15]With respect to beliefs having to do with blood, semen, bone, and male superiority I believe it would be possible to show that such beliefs have a much wider distribution throughout all of Melanesia. Certainly similarities can be found in the Solomons, the New Hebrides, New Britain, and quite likely in aboriginal Fiji.

different areas, creating different leadership patterns and differences in social structure (1987). These changes, and I think the differences are not as great as Feil claims, appear not to have affected the basic beliefs as much as one might suspect. Women in Mount Hagen are not that much better off than their Eastern Highlands counterparts when it comes to rank and status. And even in the matrilineal groups it is still mother's brother who exercises authority and is linked in some mysterious masculine fashion to sister's son. Perhaps there was less emphasis on warfare as Feil claims, but certainly there was a great deal of violence and fighting which, in fact, has broken out again in recent years.

Male initiations, particularly those employing the harshest of trials, would appear to require a climate of violence and warfare to appear and continue. If as Feil claims, there are none in parts of the Western Highlands, it is no doubt due, as he suggests, to their greater preoccupation with exchange, *moka,* and the *tee,* rather than with warring.[16] When the necessity for warfare disappeared so did the initiations. This is what happened with the Gahuku-Gama (Read 1952), the Baruya (Godelier 1986), and the Sambia (Herdt 1982). But this did not necessarily affect the underlying beliefs about the nature of men and women, bone and blood, or death and regeneration.

These beliefs may be changing, especially now after so many years of European contact, but they are changing much more slowly than did the initiation rites. The belief in the superiority of males continues. The fact that New Guinea women gained somewhat more legal rights after European contact (and that European women are gaining more presently) did not make them equal to men in ideological terms. As La Barre attempted to show, ". . . the concept of brain-*muelos* as the source of semen is everywhere inherent in European thinking,

[16]It is also quite possible that childrearing practices in the Western Highlands were such that males were indoctrinated into violence without the necessity for initiation rites as such.

as well as that of societies elsewhere" (1984:3). Even if the belief that semen comes specifically from the brain is not true everywhere, it would seem that beliefs about the importance of semen and the possibility of its depletion were or are widespread indeed.

References

Allen, M. R. 1967. *Male Cults and Secret Initiations in Melanesia.* Melbourne: Melbourne University Press.

Allen, M. R. 1984. Homosexuality, Male Power, and Political Organization in North Vanuatu: A Comparative Analysis. In *Ritualized Homosexuality in Melanesia.* G. H. Herdt (ed.). Berkeley: University of California Press, pp. 83–127.

Barlow, K. and D. Lipset 1990. Transformations of Male and Female in Murik Outrigger Canoes. Manuscript.

Barnes, J. A. 1962. African Models in the New Guinea Highlands. *Man,* 62:5–9.

Barth, F. 1975. *Ritual and Knowledge Among the Baktaman of New Guinea.* New Haven: Yale University Press.

Barth, F. 1987. *Cosmologies in the Making.* Cambridge University Press.

Barth, F. and O. Reitan 1980. Baktamin (Faiwolmin) Kinship: A Preliminary Sketch. In *Blood and Semen,* E. A. Cook and D. O'Brien (eds.). Ann Arbor University of Michigan Press, pp. 283–298.

Bateson, G. 1932. Social Structure of the Iatmul People of the Sepik River. *Oceania,* Vol. II, No. 3, pp. 245–291; 401–453.

Battaglia, D. 1985. "We Feed Our Father": Paternal Nurture Among the Sabarl of Papua New Guinea. *American Ethnologist,* Vol. 12, No. 3, pp. 427–441.

Beaver W. N. 1920. *Unexplored New Guinea.* London: Seeley, Service and Co., Ltd.

Berg, C. 1951. *The Unconscious Significance of Hair.* London.

Berndt, R. M. 1962. *Excess and Restraint.* Chicago: University of Chicago Press.

Berndt, R. M. 1964. Warfare in the New Guinea Highlands. *American Anthropologist,* Part 2, Vol. 66, No. 4, pp. 183–203.

Berndt, R. M. 1965. The Kamano, Usurufa, Jate and Fore of the Eastern

Highlands. In *Gods, Ghosts and Men in Melanesia,* P. Lawrence and M. J. Meggitt (eds.). Melbourne: Oxford University Press.

Berndt, R. M. 1992. Into the Unknown. In *Ethnographic Presents,* T. E. Hays (ed.). Berkeley: University of California Press, pp. 68–97.

Bettelheim, B. 1954. *Symbolic Wounds.* Glencoe: The Free Press.

Biersack, A. 1982. Ginger Gardens for the Ginger Woman: Rites and Passages in a Melanesian Society. *Man,* 17:239–58.

Biersack, A. 1983. Bound Blood: Paiela "Conception" Theory Interpreted. *Mankind,* Vol. 14, No. 2, pp. 85–100.

Biersack, A. 1984. Paiela "Women-Men": The Reflexive Foundations of Gender Ideology. *American Ethnologist,* Vol. 11, No. 1, pp. 118–138.

Bjerre, J. 1957. *The Last Cannibals.* New York: William Morrow and Co.

Blackwood, B. 1978. *The Kukukuku of the Upper Watut,* Monograph series, Pitt Rivers Museum, Oxford (edited by C. R. Hallpike).

Bohm, K. 1983. *The Life of Some Island People of New Guinea.* Berlin: Dietrich Reimer Verlag.

Brandewie, E. 1981. *Contrast and Context in New Guinea Culture: The Case of the Mbowamb of the Central Highlands.* Studia Instituti Anthropos, Vol. 39. St. Augustin: Anthropos Institute.

Briffault, R. 1927. *The Mothers: A Study of the Origins of Sentiments and Institutions.* New York: Macmillan.

Brongersma, L. D. and G. F. Venema. 1963. *To the Mountains of the Stars.* New York: Doubleday and Co.

Broude, G. J. 1988. Rethinking the Couvade: Cross Cultural Evidence. *American Anthropologist,* Vol. 90, No. 4, pp. 902–911.

Brown, P. 1963. From Anarchy to Satrapy. *American Anthropologist,* Vol. 65: 1–15.

Brown, P. 1969. Marriage in Chimbu. In *Pigs, Pearlshells, and Women,* R. M. Glasse and M. J. Meggitt (eds.). Englewood Cliffs, New Jersey: Prentice-Hall.

Brown, P. and G. Buchbinder (eds.) 1976. *Man and Woman in the New Guinea Highlands.* Washington: American Anthropological Association.

Bryk, F. 1934. *Circumcision in Man and Woman: Its History, Psychology and Ethnology.* American Ethnological Press.

Buchbinder, G. and R. A. Rappaport 1976. Fertility and Death Among the Maring. In *Man and Woman in the New Guinea Highlands,* P. Brown and G. Buchbinder (eds.). Washington: American Anthropological Association.

Burridge, K. 1969. *Tangu Traditions.* Oxford University Press.

Burton, R. V. and J. W. M. Whiting 1961. The Absent Father and Cross-sex Identity. *Merrill-Palmer Quarterly* 7:85–95.

Chernela, J. M. 1991. Symbolic Inaction in Rituals of Gender and Procreation among the Garifuna (Black Caribs) of Honduras. *Ethos,* Vol. 19, No. 1, pp. 52–67.

Chowning, A. 1987. Women, Exchange and Prestige in Kove. In *Dealing with Inequality*, M. Strathern (ed.). Cambridge University Press, pp. 130–149.

Clay, B. J. 1975. *Pinikindu.* Chicago: University of Chicago Press.

Codrington, R. H. 1969. *The Melanesians.* Oxford: The Clarendon Press (first published 1891).

Cohen, Y. 1964. *The Transition from Childhood to Adolescence.* Chicago: Aldine.

Collier, J. F. and M. Z. Rosaldo 1981. Politics and Gender in Simple Societies. In *Sexual Meanings: The Cultural Construction of Gender and Sexuality*, Sherry B. Ortner and Harriet Whitehead (eds.). Cambridge University Press, pp. 275–328.

Connolly, B. and R. Anderson 1987. *First Contact: New Guinea's Highlanders Encounter the Outside World.* New York: Penguin.

Cook, E. A. 1969. Marriage Among the Manga. In *Pigs, Pearlshells, and Women*, R. M. Glasse and M. J. Meggitt (eds.). Englewood Cliffs, New Jersey: Prentice-Hall.

Crapanzano, V. 1982. Rite of Return: Circumcision in Morocco. *The Psychoanalytic Study of Society*, IX:15–36.

Crawley, E. 1927. *The Mystic Rose.* New York: Boni and Liveright.

Dupeyrat, A. 1954. *Savage Papua.* New York: E. P. Dutton and Co.

Du Toit, B. M. 1975. *Akuna: A New Guinea Village Community.* Rotterdam: A. A. Balkema.

Errington, F. K. 1974. *Karavar: Masks and Power in a Melanesian Ritual.* Ithaca: Cornell University Press.

Errington, F. K. and D. Gewertz 1987. *Cultural Alternatives and a Feminist Anthropology.* Cambridge University Press.

Faithorn, E. 1976. Women as Persons. In *Man and Woman in the New Guinea Highlands*, P. Brown and G. Buchbinder (eds.). Washington: American Anthropological Association.

Feachem, R. 1973. The Religious Belief and Ritual of the Raiapu Enga. *Oceania*, Vol. XLIII, No. 4, pp. 259–285.

Feil, D. K. 1987. *The Evolution of Highland Papua New Guinea Societies.* Cambridge University Press.

Fergie, D. 1995. Transforming Women: Being and Becoming in an Island Melanesian Society. In *Gender Rituals: Female Initiation in Melanesia*, N. C. Lutkehaus and P. B. Roscoe (eds.). Routledge, pp. 113–130.

Firth, R. 1963 (1936). *We, The Tikopia.* Boston: Beacon Press.

Forge, A. 1966. Art and Environment in the Sepik. *Proceedings of the Royal Anthropological Institute for 1965*, pp. 23–32.

Fortune, R. F. 1932. *Sorcerers of Dobu.* London: George Routledge and Sons.

Fortune, R. F. 1947. The Rules of Relationship Behaviour in One Variety of Primitive Warfare. *Man*, Vol. 47, Nos. 114,115:108–110.

Frazer, J. G. 1904. The Origin of Circumcision. *Independent Review*, 4:204–218.

Freeman, D. 1979. Severed Heads that Germinate. In *Fantasy and Symbol*, R. H. Hook (ed.). London: Academic Press, pp. 233–246.

Freud, S. (1931) 1968. Female Sexuality. *The Standard Edition of the Complete Psychological Works of Sigmund Freud,* Vol. 21.

Freud, S. 1939. *Moses and Monotheism.* New York: Vintage.

Gairdner, D. 1949. The Fate of the Foreskin. *British Medical Journal,* Dec. 24, pps. 1433–1437.

Gardner, R. and K. G. Heider 1968. *Gardens of War.* New York: Random House.

Gelber, M. G. 1986. *Gender and Society in the New Guinea Highlands.* Boulder: Westview Press.

Gell, A. 1975. *Metamorphosis of the Cassowaries.* University of London: The Athlone Press.

Gillison, G. 1980. Images of Nature in Gimi Thought. In *Nature, Culture and Gender,* C. MacCormack and M. Strathern (eds.). Cambridge University Press, pp. 143–173.

Gillison, G. 1993. *Between Culture and Fantasy: A New Guinea Highlands Mythology.* Chicago: University of Chicago Press.

Glass, P. 1996. Oedipal or Tudavan? The Trobriand Nuclear Complex Revisited. *Canberra Anthropology,* 19(1), pp. 52–104.

Glasse, R. M. 1968. *Huli of Papua.* The Hague: Mouton and Co.

Glasse, R. M. 1969. Marriage in South Fore. In *Pigs, Pearlshells, and Women,* R. M. Glasse and M. J. Meggitt (eds.). Englewood Cliffs, NJ: Prentice-Hall.

Glick, L. 1963. Foundations of a Primitive Medical System: The Gimi of the New Guinea Highlands. Unpublished Ph.D. dissertation. Graduate School of Arts and Sciences, The University of Pennsylvania.

Godelier, M. 1986. *The Making of Great Men: Male Domination and Power.* Cambridge University Press.

Godelier, M. 1989. Betrayal: The Case of the New Guinea Baruya. *Oceania,* Vol. 59, No. 3, pp. 165–180.

Graber, R. B. 1981. A Psychocultural Theory of Male Genital Mutilation. *The Journal of Psychoanalytic Anthropology,* 4:4:413–434.

Gray, B. M. 1982. Enga Birth, Maturation and Survival: Physiological Characteristics of the Life Cycle in the New Guinea Highlands. In *Ethnography of Fertility and Birth,* C. P. MacCormack (ed.). Academic Press, pp. 75–113.

Haddon, A. C. 1904. Funeral Ceremonies. In *Reports of the Cambridge Anthropological Expedition to Torres Straits,* Vol. 5, pp. 248–262.

Hallpike, C. R. 1977. *Bloodshed and Vengeance in the Papuan Mountains.* Oxford: The Clarendon Press.

Harrington. C. 1968. Sexual Differentiation in Socialization and Some Male Genital Mutilations. *American Anthropologist,* 70:5:951–956.

Hauser-Schaublin, B. 1995. Puberty Rites, Women's *Naven,* and Initiation: Women's Rituals of Transition in Abelam and Iatmul Culture. In *Gender Rituals: Female Initiation in Melanesia,* N. C. Lutkehaus and P. B. Roscoe (eds.). New York and London: Routledge.

Hawkins, M. 1984. Gender Symbolism and Power Relations: A Reassessment of the *Amb Kor* Cult of Mt. Hagen. *Mankind,* Vol. 14, No. 3, pp. 217–224.

Hays. T. E. 1986. Sacred Flutes, Fertility, and Growth in the Papua New Guinea Highlands. *Anthropos,* 81:435–453.

Hays, T. E. 1987. Initiation as Experience. In *Anthropology in the High Valleys,* L. L. Langness and T. E. Hays (eds.). Novato, California: Chandler & Sharp.

Hays, T. E. 1988. "Myths of Matriarchy" and the Sacred Flute Complex of the Papua New Guinea Highlands. In *Myths of Matriarchy Reconsidered,* Deborah Gewertz (ed.). Oceania Monograph No. 33, pp. 98–120.

Hays, T. E. 1992. A Historical Background to Anthropology in the Papua New Guinea Highlands. In *Ethnographic Presents,* T. E. Hays (ed.). Berkeley: University of California Press, pp. 1–36.

Hays, T. E. 1993. The New Guinea Highlands. *Current Anthropology,* Vol. 13, No. 2, pp. 141–164.

Hays, T. E. 1994. Personal communication.

Hays, T. E. and P. Hays 1982. Opposition and Complementarity of the Sexes in Ndumba Initiation. In *Rituals of Manhood: Male Initiation in Papua New Guinea,* G. H. Herdt (ed.). Berkeley: University of California Press, pp. 201–238.

Heider, K. G. 1970. *The Dugum Dani.* Chicago: Aldine.

Heider, K. G. 1976. Dani Sexuality: A Low Energy System. *Man,* Vol. 11, No. 2, pp. 188–201.

Held, G. J. 1957. *The Papuans of Waropen.* The Hague: Martinus Nijhoff.

Herdt, G. H. 1981. *Guardians of the Flutes.* New York: McGraw-Hill.

Herdt, G. H. (ed.) 1982. *Rituals of Manhood: Male Initiation in Papua New Guinea.* Berkeley: University of California Press.

Herdt, G. H. 1982a. Fetish and Fantasy in Sambia Initiation. In *Rituals of Manhood: Male Initiation in Papua New Guinea,* G. H. Herdt (ed.). Berkeley: University of California Press, pp. 44–98.

Herdt, G. H. 1982b. Sambia Nosebleeding Rites and Male Proximity to Women. *Ethos,* Vol. 10, No. 3, pp. 189–231.

Herdt, G. H. (ed.) 1984. *Ritualized Homosexuality in Melanesia.* Berkeley: University of California Press.

Herdt, G. H. 1984a. Semen Transactions in Sambia Culture. In *Ritualized Homosexuality in Melanesia,* G. H. Herdt (ed.). Berkeley: University of California Press.

Herdt, G. H. 1984b. Ritualized Homosexual Behavior in the Male Cults of Melanesia, 1862–1983: An Introduction. In *Ritualized Homosexuality in Melanesia,* G. H. Herdt (ed.). Berkeley: University of California Press, pp. 1–82.

Herdt, G. H. 1989. Father Presence and Ritual Homosexuality: Paternal Deprivation and Masculine Development in Melanesia Reconsidered. *Ethos,* Vol. 17, No. 3, pp 326–370.

Herdt, G. H. 1990. The Causes of Homosexuality: An Essay on Cultural Ontology and Historical Comparison. Manuscript.

Herdt, G. H. 1990a. Secret Societies and Secret Collectives. *Oceania,* Vol. 60, No. 4, pp. 361–381.

Herdt, G. H., and M. Stephen 1989. *The Religious Imagination in New Guinea.* New Brunswick: Rutgers University Press.

Herdt, G. H., and R. J. Stoller 1990. *Intimate Communications.* New York: Columbia University Press.

Hiatt, L. R. 1971. Secret Pseudo-procreation Rites Among the Australian Aborigines. In *Anthroplogy in Oceania: Essays Presented to Ian Hogbin,* L. R. Hiatt and C. Jayawardena (eds.). Sydney: Angus and Robertson, pp. 77–88.

Hides, J. G. 1935. *Through Wildest Papua.* London: Blackie and Sons.

Hogbin, I. 1970. *The Island of Menstruating Men.* Scranton: Chandler Publishing Company.

Hollan, D. and J. Wellenkamp 1990. *Contentment and Suffering.* Manuscript.

Honigmann, J. 1967. *Personality in Culture.* New York: Harper and Row.

Hutton, J. H. 1928. The Significance of Head-hunting in Assam. *Journal of the Royal Anthropological Institute,* 58:399–408.

Ivens, W. G. 1927. *Melenesians of the South-east Solomon Islands.* New York: Benjamin Blom, Inc.

Jacobson, E. 1950. Development of the Wish for a Child in Boys. *The Psychoanalytic Study of the Child,* Vol. 5, p. 142.

Jensen. E. 1974. *The Iban and Their Religion.* Oxford: Clarendon Press.

Jorgensen, D. 1983. The Facts of Life, Papua New Guinea Style. *Mankind,* Vol. 14, No. 1, pp. 1–12.

Jorgensen, D. 1983a. Mirroring Nature? Men's and Women's Models of Conception in Telefolmin. *Mankind,* Vol. 14, No. 1, pp. 57–65.

Juillerat, B. (ed.) 1992. *Shooting the Sun: Ritual and Meaning in West Sepik.* Washington: Smithsonian Institute Press.

Jung, C. 1972. *Collected Works,* Vol. 7, *Two Essays on Analytical Psychology.* Princeton: Princeton University Press.

Kaberry, P. M. 1941. The Abelam Tribe, Sepik District, New Guinea. *Oceania,* Vol. XI, No. 3, pp. 233–258.

Kaberry, P. M. 1941a. The Abelam Tribe, Sepik District, New Guinea: A Preliminary Report. *Oceania,* Vol. XI, No. 4, pp. 345–367.

Kaberry, P. M. 1971. Political Organization Among the Northern Abelam. In *Politics in New Guinea,* R. M. Berndt and P. Lawrence (eds.). University of Western Australia Press, pp. 35–66.

Keesing, R. 1985. Conventional Metaphors and Anthropological Metaphysics: The Problematic of Cultural Translation. *Journal of Anthropological Research,* Vol. 41, No. 2, pp. 201–218.

Keesing, R. 1987. Ta'a geni: Women's Perspectives on Kwaio Society. In *Dealing with Inequality,* M. Strathern (ed.). Cambridge University Press, pp. 33–62.

Kelly, R. C. 1976. Witchcraft and Sexual Relations. In *Man and Woman in the New Guinea Highlands*, P. Brown and G. Buchbinder (eds.). Washington: American Anthropological Association.

Kelly, R. C. 1977. *Etoro Social Structure.* Ann Arbor: University of Michigan Press.

Kelly, R. C. 1993. *Constructing Inequality.* Ann Arbor: University of Michigan Press.

Kennedy, J. G. 1970. Circumcision and Excision in Egyptian Nubia. *Man*, Vol. 5 (n.s.): 175–191.

Knauft, B. M. 1985. *Good Company and Violence.* Berkeley: University of California Press.

Knauft, B. M. 1986. Text and Social Practice: Narrative "Longing" and Bixexuality Among the Gebusi of New Guinea. *Ethos*, Vol. 14, No. 3, pp. 252–281.

Knauft, B. M. 1990. Melanesian Warfare: A Theoretical History. *Oceania*, Vol. 60, No. 4, pp. 250–311.

Koch, K. 1974. *War and Peace in Jalemo.* Harvard University Press.

Koch, K. 1974a. Sociogenic and Psychogenic Models in Anthropology: The Functions of Jale Initiation. *Man*, Vol. 9, No. 3, pp. 397–422.

Kurtz, S. N. 1991. Polysexualization: A New Approach to Oedipus in the Trobriands. *Ethos*, Vol. 19, No. 1, pp. 68–101.

Kurtz, S. N. 1993. A Trobriand Complex. *Ethos*, Vol. 21, No. 1, pp. 79–103.

La Barre, W. 1984. *Muelos.* New York: Columbia University Press.

La Fontaine, J. 1978. The Power of Rights. *Man*, 12:421–437.

Landtman, G. 1927. *The Kiwai Papuans of British New Guinea.* London: Macmillan.

Langness, L. L. 1963. Notes on the Bena Council, Eastern Highlands. *Oceania*, XXXIII, No. 3, pp. 153–70.

Langness, L. L. 1965. Hysterical Psychosis in the New Guinea Highlands: A Bena Bena Example. *Psychiatry*, 28:259–277.

Langness, L. L. 1967. Sexual Antagonism in the New Guinea Highlands: A Bena Bena Example. *Oceania*, 37:161–177.

Langness, L. L. 1969. Marriage in Bena Bena. In *Pigs, Pearlshells, and Women*, R. M. Glasse and M. J. Meggitt (eds.). New York: Prentice Hall.

Langness, L. L. 1972. Violence in the New Guinea Highlands. In *The Illumination of Collective Violence*, J. F. Short and M. E. Wolfgang (eds.). New York: Aldine.

Langness, L. L. 1972a. Political Organization. In *The Encyclopedia of Papua New Guinea*, P. Ryan (ed.). Melbourne: Melbourne University Press, pp. 922–934.

Langness, L. L. 1974. Ritual, Power and Male Dominance in the New Guinea Highlands. *Ethos*, 2:182–212.

Langness, L. L. 1976. The Nupasafa Cattle: Rural Development in the New Guinea Highlands. In *New Guinea Research Bulletin*, No. 63, pp. 67–90.

Langness, L. L. 1981. Child Abuse and Cultural Values: The Case of New

Guinea. In *Child Abuse and Neglect: A Cross-Cultural Perspective,* J. E. Korbin (ed.). Berkeley: University of California Press.

Langness, L. L. and T. Hays (eds.) 1987. *Anthropology in the High Valleys.* Novato, California: Chandler & Sharp.

Lattas, A. 1990. Poetics of Space and Sexual Economies of Power: Gender and the Politics of Male Identity in West New Britain. *Ethos,* 18:1, 71–102.

Lawrence, P. 1971. The Garia of the Madang District. In *Politics in New Guinea,* R. M. Berndt and P. Lawrence (eds.). University of Western Australia Press, pp. 74–91.

Lawrence, P. 1984. *The Garia.* Melbourne University Press.

Lawrence, P. and M. J. Meggitt 1965. *Gods, Ghosts and Men in Melanesia.* Melbourne: Oxford University Press.

Layard, J. 1942. *Stone Men of Malekula.* London: Chatto and Windus.

Leach. E. 1958. Magical Hair. *The Journal of the Royal Anthropological Institute of Great Britain and Ireland,* Vol. 88, Part II, pp. 147–164.

Leavitt, S. C. 1991. Sexual Ideology and Experience in a Papua New Guinea Society. *Social Science and Medicine,* Vol. 33, No. 8, pp. 897–907.

Leininger, M. 1966. *Convergence and Divergence of Human Behavior: An Ethnopsychological Comparative Study of Two Gadsup Villages in the Eastern Highlands of New Guinea.* Ph.D. dissertation, University of Washington.

LeTourneau, C. 1893. De l'origine de la circoncision chez les Juifs. *Bulletin de la Societe d'Anthropologies de Paris.* pp. 208–210.

Levy, R. I. 1973. *Tahitians.* Chicago: University of Chicago Press.

Lewis, G. 1975. *Knowledge of Illness in a Sepik Society.* London School of Economics Monographs on Social Anthropology No. 52.

Lewis, G. 1980. *Day of Shining Red.* Cambridge University Press.

Lewis, I. M. 1966. Spirit Possession and Deprivation Cults. *Man,* I, 307–330.

Leys, S. 1995. Balzac's Genius and Other Paradoxes. *The New York Review of Books,* Vol. XLII, No. 1, pp. 22–24.

Lidz, T. and R. W. 1989. *Oedipus in the Stone Age.* Madison, Connecticut: International Universities Press, Inc.

Lindenbaum, S. 1976. A Wife is the Hand of Man. In *Man and Woman in the New Guinea Highlands,* P. Brown and G. Buchbinder (eds.). Special Publication of the American Anthropological Association, No. 8.

Lindenbaum, S. 1979. *Kuru Sorcery.* Mayfield Publishing Company.

Lipset, D. n.d. Food, Vines and Canoes. Manuscript.

Lipset, D. n.d. Mwara Yakabor: The Trickster/Guardians of the Threshold. Manuscript.

Loving, R. 1974. Notes on Awa Kinship Terminology. In *Kinship Studies in Papua New Guinea,* D. Shaw (ed.). Ukarumpa: SIL Press, pp. 115–24.

Lowman-Vayda, C. 1968. "Maring Big Men." *Anthropological Forum,* pp. 199–243.

Luhrmann, T. M. 1989. The Magic of Secrecy. *Ethos,* Vol. 17, No. 2, pp. 131–165.

Lutkehaus, N. C. 1995. Feminist Anthropology and Female Initiation in Melanesia. In *Gender Rituals: Female Initiation in Melanesia,* N. C. Lutkehaus and P. B. Roscoe (eds.). New York and London: Routledge.

Lutkehaus, N. C. and P. B. Roscoe (eds.) 1995. *Gender Rituals: Female Initiation in Melanesia,* New York and London: Routledge.

MacCormack, C., and M. Strathern (eds.) 1980. *Nature, Culture and Gender.* Cambridge University Press.

Malcolm, L. A. 1966. The Age of Puberty in the Bundi People. *Papua New Guinea Medical Journal,* 9:I:16.

Malcolm, L. A. 1970. Growth and Development in New Guinea—A Study of the Bundi People of the Madang District. Monograph Series Number l, Institute of Human Biology, Madang.

Malcolm, L. A. 1970a. Growth, Malnutrition, and Mortality of the Infant and Toddler in the Asai Valley of the New Guinea Highlands. *The American Journal of Clinical Nutrition,* 23:8:1090–1095.

Malinowski, B. 1922. *Argonauts of the Western Pacific.* New York: E. P. Dutton.

Malinowski, B. 1929. *The Sexual Life of Savages in North-Western Melanesia.* New York: Harcourt, Brace and World.

Mandeville, E. 1979. Agnation, Affinity and Migration Among the Kamano of the New Guinea Highlands. *Man* (n.s.) 14:105–23.

Matthiessen, P. 1962. *Under the Mountain Wall.* New York: Viking Press.

Mbaginta'o, I. 1971. The Anga Initiations. *Journal Society des Oceanistes,* 27:32, pp. 285–294.

McCarthy, J. K. 1963. *Patrol into Yesterday.* Sydney: F. W. Cheshire.

Mead, M. 1935. *Sex and Temperament.* New York: Morrow.

Mead, M. 1938. *The Mountain Arapesh: I. An Importing Culture.* Anthropological Papers of the American Museum of Natural History, Vol. XXXVI, Part III, pp. 139–349.

Mead, M. 1940–41. *The Mountain Arapesh: II. Supernaturalism.* Anthropological Papers of the American Museum of Natural History, Vol. XXXVII, Part III, pp. 317–451.

Meeker, M. E., K. Barlow and D. M. Lipset 1986. Culture, Exchange, and Gender: Lessons from the Murik. *Cultural Anthropology,* 1:1:6–73.

Meggitt, M. J. 1964. Male-Female Relationships in the Highlands of Australian New Guinea. In *New Guinea The Central Highlands,* J. B. Watson (ed.). Special Publication of the American Anthropological Association (*American Anthropologist,* Part 2, Volume 66, Number 4).

Meggitt, M. J. 1965. *The Mae-Enga of the New Guinea Highlands.* New York: Barnes and Noble.

Meggitt, M. J. 1977. *Blood is Their Argument.* Mayfield Publishing Company.

Meigs, A. S. 1976. Male Pregnancy and the Reduction of Sexual Opposition in a New Guinea Highlands Society. *Ethnology,* Vol. XV, No. 4, pp. 393–408.

Meigs, A. S. 1984. *Food, Sex, and Pollution.* New Brunswick: Rutgers University Press.

Miklouho-Maclay, N. 1982. *Travels to New Guinea.* London: Progress Publishers.

Morgan, L. H. 1877. *Ancient Society.* New York: World Publishing.

Mosco, M. S. 1983. Conception, Deconception and Social Structure in Bush Mekeo Culture. *Mankind,* Vol. 14, pp. 24–32.

Mytinger, C. 1942. *Headhunting in the Solomon Islands.* New York: MacMillan.

Newman, P. 1965. *Knowing the Gururumba.* New York: Holt, Rinehart and Winston.

Newman, P. 1981. Sexual Politics and Witchcraft in Two New Guinea Societies. In *Social Inequality: Comparative and Developmental Approaches,* Gerald D. Berreman (ed.). New York: Academic Press, pp. 103–121.

Newman, P. 1989. Personal communication.

Newman, P., and D. Boyd 1982. The Making of Men. In *Rituals of Manhood: Male Initiation in Papua New Guinea,* G. Herdt (ed.). Berkeley: University of California Press.

Nilles, J. 1950. The Kuman of the Chimbu Region, Central Highlands, New Guinea. *Oceania,* XXI, No. 1, pp. 25–65.

Norbeck, E., Donald E. Walker, and Mimi Cohen 1962. The Interpretation of Data: Puberty Rites. *American Anthropologist,* 64: 463–485

O'Hanlon, M., and L. Frankland 1986. With a Skull in the Netbag: Prescriptive Marriage and Matrilateral Relations in the New Guinea Highlands. *Oceania,* 56:3:181–198.

Ortner, S. 1974. Is Female to Male as Nature is to Culture? In *Woman, Culture, and Society,* M. Z. Rosaldo and L. Lamphere (eds.). Stanford University Press, pp. 67–87.

Oster, J. 1968. Further Fate of the Foreskin. *Archives of Disease in Childhood,* April, pps. 200–202.

Parker, S., J. Smith, and J. Ginat 1975. Father Absence and Cross-Sex Identity: The Puberty Rites Controversy Revisited. *American Ethnologist,* Vol. 2, No. 4, pp. 687–706.

Poole, F. J. P. 1975. *WANENG AIYEM*: "Sacred" and "Polluting" Dimensions of Female Identity in Bimin-Kuskusmin Society. Paper read at the 74th Annual Meeting of the American Anthropological Association, San Francisco, 41 pages.

Poole, F. J. P. 1981. Female Ritual Leaders Among Bimin-Kuskusmin. In *Sexual Meanings,* S. B. Ortner and H. Whitehead (eds.). Cambridge University Press, pp. 116–165.

Poole, F. J. P. 1982. The Ritual Forging of Identity. In *Rituals of Manhood: Male Initiation in Papua New Guinea,* G. Herdt (ed.). Berkeley: University of California Press.

Poole, F. J. P. 1984. Symbols of Substance: Bimin-Kuskusmin Models of Procreation, Death and Personhood. *Mankind,* Vol. 14, No. 3, pp. 191–216.

Pospisil, L. 1958. *Kapauku Papuans and their Law.* Yale Publications in Anthropology, No. 54. New Haven: Yale University Press.

Pospisil, L. 1964. *Kapauku Papuans and Their Law.* New Haven: Human Relations Area Files Press.

Powdermaker, H. 1971. *Life in Lesu.* New York: W. W. Norton & Co.

Rappaport, R. A. 1968. *Pigs for the Ancestors.* New Haven: Yale University Press.

Read, K. E. 1952. Nama Cult of the Central Highlands, New Guinea. *Oceania,* Vol. 23, No. 1, pp. 1–25.

Read, K. E. 1954. Marriage Among the Gahuku-Gama of the Eastern Central Highlands, New Guinea. *South Pacific,* Vol. 7, No. 10, pp. 864–871.

Read, K. E. 1955. Morality and the Concept of the Person Among the Gahuku-Gama, Eastern Highlands, New Guinea. *Oceania,* Vol. 25, No. 4, pp. 233–282.

Read, K. E. 1959. Leadership and Consensus in a New Guinea Society. *American Anthropologist,* Vol. 61, No. 3, pp. 425–436.

Read, K. E. 1965. *The High Valley.* New York: Charles Scribner's Sons.

Read, K. E. 1982. Male-Female Relationships Among the Gahuku-Gama: 1950 and 1981. In *Sexual Antagonism, Gender, and Social Change in Papua New Guinea,* F. J. P. Poole and G. H. Herdt (eds.). Special Issue *Social Analysis,* No. 12.

Read, K. E. 1986. *Return to the High Valley.* Berkeley: University of California Press.

Reay, M. 1959. *The Kuma.* Melbourne: Melbourne University Press.

Reay, M. 1992. An Innocent in the Garden of Eden. In *Ethnographic Presents,* Terence E. Hays (ed.). Berkeley: University of California Press, pp. 137–166.

Reik, T. 1975. *Ritual: Psychoanalytic Studies.* Douglas Brylan, trans. Westport: Greenwood Press.

Robbins, S. 1982. *Auyana: Those Who Held onto Home.* Seattle: University of Washington Press.

Roscoe, P. B. 1994. Amity and Aggression: A Symbolic Theory of Incest. *Man,* Vol. 29, No. 1, pp. 49–76.

Roscoe, P. B. 1995. In the Shadow of the Tambaran: Female Initiation Among the Ndu of the Sepik Basin. In *Gender Rituals: Female Initiation in Melanesia,* N. C. Lutkehaus and P. B. Roscoe (eds.). Routledge, pp. 55–84.

Ryan, D. 1969. Marriage in Mendi. In *Pigs, Pearlshells, and Women,* R. M. Glasse and M. J. Meggitt (eds.). Englewood Cliffs, NJ: Prentice-Hall.

Ryder, L. 1989. Personal communication.

Salisbury, R. F. 1962. *From Stone to Steel.* Melbourne University Press.

Salisbury, R. F. 1965. The Siane of the Eastern Highlands. In *Gods, Ghosts and Men in Melanesia,* P. Lawrence and M. J. Meggitt (eds.). Oxford University Press.

Saulnier, T. 1963. *Headhunters of Papua.* New York: Crown Publishers.

Schieffelin, B. B. 1990. *The Give and Take of Everyday Life.* Cambridge University Press.

Schieffelin, E. L. 1976. *The Sorrow of the Lonely and the Burning of the Dancers.* New York: St. Martin's Press.

Schieffelin, E. L. and R. Crittenden, et al. 1991. *Like People You See in a Dream.* Stanford University Press.

Schwimmer, E. G. 1969. Letter on Virgin Birth. *Man,* (n.s.), 4:132–3.

Schwimmer, E. G. 1974. Object of Mediation: Myth and Praxis. In *The Unconscious in Culture,* I. Rossi (ed.). pp. 209–237. New York: Dutton.

Schwimmer, E. G. 1984. Male Couples in New Guinea. In *Ritualized Homosexuality in Melanesia,* G. H. Herdt (ed.). Berkeley: University of California Press, pp. 248–291.

Serpenti, L. M. 1965. *Cultivators in the Swamps.* Assen: Van Gorcum and Co.

Serpenti, L. M. 1984. Ritual Homosexuality and Pedophilia Among Kimam-Papuans. In *Ritualized Homosexuality in Melanesia,* G. H. Herdt (ed.). Berkeley: University of California Press, pp. 292–317.

Shweder, R. A. 1984. Anthropology's Romantic Rebellion Against the Enlightenment, or There's More to Thinking than Reason and Evidence. In *Culture Theory,* R. A. Shweder and R. A. LeVine (eds.). Cambridge University Press, pp. 27–66.

Simpson, C. 1953. *Adam with Arrows.* Sydney: Angus and Robertson.

Simpson, C. 1954. *Adam in Plumes.* Sydney: Angus and Robertson.

Sinclair, J. P. 1966. *Behind the Ranges.* Melbourne: Melbourne University Press.

Sinnett, P. 1971. Nutrition in a New Guinea Highland Community. *Human Biology in Oceania,* 1:4:299–305.

Sinnett, P., and H. M. Whyte 1973. Epidemiological Studies in a Highland Population of New Guinea: Environment, Culture and Health Status. *Human Ecology,* 1:3:270.

Sorum, A. 1982. The Seeds of Power: Patterns in Bedamini Male Initiation. *Social Analysis,* No. 10, pp. 42–62.

Sorum, A. 1984. Growth and Decay: Bedamini Notions of Sexuality. In *Ritualized Homosexuality in Melanesia,* G. H. Herdt (ed.). Berkeley: University of California Press, pp. 318–336.

Sorenson, E. R. 1976. *The Edge of the Forest.* Smithsonian Institution Press.

Spiro, M. E. 1979. *Gender and Culture: Kibbutz Women Revisited.* Durham: Duke University Press.

Spiro, M. E. 1982. *Oedipus in the Trobriands.* Chicago: University of Chicago Press.

Spiro, M. E. 1992. Oedipus Redux. *Ethos,* Vol. 20, No. 3, pp. 358–376.

Stoller, R. J. 1975. *Perversion.* New York: Quadrangle.

Stoller, R. J. 1985. *Presentations of Gender.* New Haven: Yale University Press

Stoller, R. J. 1985a. *Observing the Erotic Imagination.* New Haven: Yale University Press.

Stoller, R. J., and G. H. Herdt 1985. Theories of Origins of Male Homosexuality. *Archives of General Psychiatry,* 42:399–404.

Stoller, R. J., and G. H. Herdt 1985a. Theories of Origins of Male Homosexuality: A Cross-Cultural Look. In *Observing the Erotic Imagination,* R. J. Stoller (ed.). New Haven: Yale University Press, pp. 104–134.

Strathern, A. 1970. The Female and Male Spirit Cults in Mount Hagen. *Man*, 5:571–585.

Strathern, A. 1971. *The Rope of Moka.* Cambridge University Press.

Strathern, A. 1972. *One Father, One Blood.* Canberra: Australian National University Press.

Strathern, A. 1996. *Body Thoughts.* Ann Arbor: University of Michigan Press.

Strathern, A., and M. Strathern 1969. Marriage in Melpa. In *Pigs, Pearlshells, and Women*, R. M. Glass and M. J. Meggitt (eds.). Englewood Cliffs, NJ: Prentice-Hall, pp. 138–158.

Strathern, M. 1978. The Achievement of Sex: Paradoxes in Hagen Gender-thinking. In *Yearbook of Symbolic Anthropology*, E. G. Schwimmer (ed.). McGill-Queens University Press/Hurst.

Strathern, M. 1988. *The Gender of the Gift.* Berkeley: University of California Press.

Tuzin, D. 1980. *The Voice of the Tambaran.* Berkeley: University of California Press.

Tuzin, D. 1982. Ritual Violence Among the Ilahita Arapesh. In *Rituals of Manhood: Male Initiation in Papua New Guinea*, G. H. Herdt (ed.). Berkeley: University of California Press, pp. 321–355.

Tuzin, D. 1987. Procreation, Parthenogenesis and Other Private Matters in the Western Pacific. Paper delivered to the 86th Annual Meeting of the American Anthropological Association, Chicago.

Van Baal, J. 1966. *Dema.* The Hague: Martinus Nÿhoff. (Current copyright holder is KITLV Press, Royal Institute of Linguistics and Anthropology, The Netherlands.)

Van Baal, J. 1984. The Dialectics of Sex in Marind-anim Culture. In *Ritualized Homosexuality in Melanesia*, G. H. Herdt (ed.). Berkeley: University of California Press, pp. 128–166.

Van Gennep, A. 1960. *The Rites of Passage.* Chicago: University of Chicago Press.

Vicedom, Georg F. and Herbert Tischner 1943–48. *Die Mbowamb: Die Kultur der Hagenberg-stamme im ostlichen Zentral-Neuguinea.* 3 vols. Hamburgischen Museum fur Volkerkunde, Monographien zur Volkerkunde no. 1. Hamburg.

Wagner, R. 1972. *Habu.* Chicago: University of Chicago Press.

Wagner, R. 1980. Daribi Kinship. In *Blood and Semen*, E. A. Cook and D. O'Brien (eds.). Ann Arbor: University of Michigan Press, pp. 423–440.

Wagner, R. 1983. The Ends of Innocence: Conception and Seduction among the Daribi of Karimui and the Barok of New Ireland. *Mankind*, Vol. 14, No. 1, pp. 75–83.

Watson, J. B. 1971. Tairora: The Politics of Despotism in a Small Society. In *Politics in New Guinea*, R. M. Berndt and P. Lawrence (eds.). University of Western Australia Press, pp. 224–287

Watson, J. B. 1983. *Tairora Culture: Contingency and Pragmatism.* Seattle: University of Washington Press.

Weiner, A. B. 1982. Sexuality Among the Anthropologists: Reproduction

Among the Informants. In *Sexual Antagonism, Gender, and Social Change in Papua New Guinea,* F. J. P. Poole and G. H. Herdt (eds.). Special Issue Series Social Analysis No. 12. Adelaide, South Australia.

Weiner, A. B. 1976. *Women of Value, Men of Renown.* Austin: University of Texas Press.

Weiner, A. B. 1985. Oedipus and Ancestors. *American Ethnologist,* Vol 12, No. 4, pp. 758–762.

Weiner, J. F. 1987. Diseases of the Soul: Sickness, Agency and the Men's Cult among the Foi of New Guinea. In *Dealing with Inequality,* M. Strathern (ed.). Cambridge University Press, pp. 255–276.

Weiner, J. F. 1988. *The Heart of the Pearl Shell.* Berkeley: University of California Press.

Weiner, J. F. 1988a (ed.). *Mountain Papuans Historical and Comparative Perspectives from New Guinea Fringe Highland Societies.* Ann Arbor: University of Michigan Press.

Weiner, J. F. 1995. *The Lost Drum The Myth of Sexuality in Papua New Guinea and Beyond.* Madison: University of Wisconsin Press.

Westermarck, E. 1926. *A Short History of Marriage.* New York: Macmillan.

Whitehead, H. 1986. The Varieties of Fertility Cultism in New Guinea: Part I. *American Ethnologist,* Vol. 13, No. 1, pp. 80–99.

Whitehead, H. 1986a. The Varieties of Fertility Cultism in New Guinea: Part II. *American Ethnologist,* Vol. 13, No. 2, pp. 271–289.

Whiting, J. W. M. 1941. *Becoming a Kwoma.* New Haven: Yale University Press.

Whiting, J. W. M., R. Kluckhohn, and A. Anthony 1958. The Function of Male Initiation Ceremonies at Puberty. In *Readings in Social Psychology,* E. E. Maccoby, T. M. Newcomb, and E. L. Hartley (eds.). New York: Henry Holt and Co.

Whiting, J. W. M. and S. W. Reed 1938. Kwoma Culture Report on Field Work in the Mandated Territory of New Guinea. *Oceania,* Vol. 9, pp. 170–216.

Willey, K. 1965. *Assignment New Guinea.* Brisbane: The Jacaranda Press.

Williams, F. E. 1930. *Okokaiva Society.* Oxford: Clarendon Press.

Williams, F. E. 1936. *Papuans of the Trans-Fly.* London: Oxford University Press.

Williams, F. E. 1940. *Natives of Lake Kutubu, Papua.* Oceania Monograph No. 6. Sydney.

Wright, M. 1966. *The Gentle Savage.* Melbourne: Landsdowne Press.

Young, F. 1962. The Function of Male Initiation Ceremonies: A Cross-cultural Test of an Alternative Hypothesis. *American Journal of Sociology,* 67:379–391.

Index